Patient-Centered Health Education

Patient-Centered Health Education

UNDERSTANDING STAGES OF CHANGE

Jessica Alicea

Fairfield University

cognella®
SAN DIEGO

Bassim Hamadeh, CEO and Publisher
Amanda Martin, Executive Publisher
Alverne Ball, Project Editor
Rachel Kahn, Production Editor
Jess Estrella, Senior Graphic Designer
Laura Duncan, Licensing Specialist
Tiffany Mok, Senior Content Marketing Specialist
Natalie Piccotti, Director of Marketing
Kassie Graves, Senior Vice President, Editorial
Alia Bales, Director of Project Editorial & Production

Printed in the United States of America.

To my parents, Manny and Patty, whose love, sacrifices, and unwavering belief in me helped shape the person I am today. Thank you for believing in me and encouraging me to pursue my goals.

And to my children, Alana and Mateo, who give my life its deepest purpose and inspire me every day to become the best version of myself.

BRIEF CONTENTS

DETAILED CONTENTS

ACKNOWLEDGMENTS

I would like to express my deepest gratitude to the many patients who have allowed me the privilege of working alongside them as they strive to make meaningful changes in their health. Their trust, resilience, and willingness to share their stories have shaped not only my understanding of patient-centered care but also my growth as a nurse and educator. I am also profoundly grateful to the mentors who have guided me throughout my journey, generously offering their wisdom, encouragement, and thoughtful responses to my many questions. Finally, I would like to acknowledge the invaluable experiences I gained while working at a federally qualified health center in Bridgeport, Connecticut. The lessons learned from that community and the individuals I had the honor to serve continue to influence and inspire the work reflected in this book.

INTRODUCTION

Chronic conditions are a significant health concern in the United States, affecting millions of people and placing a substantial burden on the healthcare system. Six in 10 Americans live with at least one chronic health condition (Centers for Disease Control and Prevention [CDC], 2024a), and the number of people living with multiple chronic conditions is steadily rising among both children and adults (Multiple Chronic Conditions Resource Center [MCCRC], 2025). This patient population uses a significant amount of healthcare resources, accounting for 64% of all clinician visits, 70% of all inpatient stays, 83% of all prescriptions, 71% of all healthcare spending, and 93% of Medicare spending (MCCRC, 2025). In fact, a shocking 90% of the nation's $4.9 trillion health expenditures are for people with chronic and mental health conditions (CDC, 2024b). Therefore, interventions to prevent and manage these conditions can have substantial economic benefits, in addition to the obvious health advantages.

Following are some of the most prevalent chronic conditions in the United States:

1. **Heart disease:** Heart disease remains the leading cause of death in the United States. It encompasses a range of conditions affecting the heart and blood vessels, including coronary artery disease, heart attacks, and heart failure (National Center for Health Statistics, 2025).
2. **Diabetes:** Both type 1 and type 2 diabetes are prevalent in the United States, with type 2 diabetes being more common. Diabetes can lead to serious complications, such as cardiovascular disease, kidney failure, and blindness, if it's not properly managed. Nearly 23% of adults with diabetes living in the United States are undiagnosed (CDC, 2024c).

3. **Obesity:** Obesity is a significant risk factor for numerous chronic conditions, including heart disease, diabetes, and certain types of cancer. It has reached epidemic proportions in the United States, with approximately 42% of adults classified as obese (CDC, 2024d).
4. **Hypertension (high blood pressure):** High blood pressure is a common condition that increases the risk of heart disease, stroke, and other complications. Nearly half of U.S. adults have high blood pressure, with many cases going undiagnosed or uncontrolled (Division for Heart Disease and Stroke Prevention, 2023).
5. **Chronic respiratory diseases:** Conditions such as chronic obstructive pulmonary disease, asthma, and sleep apnea contribute to significant morbidity and mortality in the United States (NCD Alliance, n.d.). These conditions can impair lung function and quality of life.
6. **Cancer:** Cancer encompasses a diverse group of diseases characterized by the uncontrolled growth and spread of abnormal cells. It remains a leading cause of death in the United States, with lung cancer, breast cancer, prostate cancer, and colorectal cancer among the most common types (National Cancer Institute, 2025).

Addressing chronic conditions requires a multifaceted approach involving preventive measures, lifestyle modifications, access to healthcare services, and effective management strategies. Personalized health education fosters a more patient-centered approach to chronic disease management, promoting better outcomes, improved quality of life, and reduced healthcare costs in the long term. Appropriate health education can significantly enhance chronic disease management for several reasons (see Box I.1).

Box I.1 The Role of Health Education in Chronic Disease Management

Tailored information: Personalized health education can provide individuals with information that is specifically relevant to their unique health needs, preferences, and circumstances. By addressing individual concerns and challenges, individualized health education increases the likelihood that the information will be understood, remembered, and acted upon effectively.

Increased engagement: When individuals receive information that directly relates to their health status and goals, they are more likely to engage with the educational materials and take proactive steps to manage their condition. Personalization can foster a sense of relevance and ownership, motivating individuals to participate in their own care.

Improved understanding: Personalized health education can clarify complex medical concepts and treatment options by presenting information in a way that resonates with the individual's knowledge level and learning style. This facilitates better comprehension and retention of important health information, leading to more informed decision-making.

Behavioral change: Chronic disease management often requires significant lifestyle modifications, such as dietary changes, exercise routines, medication adherence, and stress management techniques. Personalized health education can provide tailored guidance and support to help individuals overcome barriers to behavior change and adopt healthier habits.

Enhanced adherence: Adherence to treatment plans is essential for effectively managing chronic conditions and preventing complications. Personalized health education can address individual concerns, misconceptions, and barriers to adherence, increasing the likelihood that individuals will follow through with their prescribed therapies and recommendations.

Empowerment: Personalized health education empowers individuals to take an active role in managing their health and well-being. By providing relevant information, resources, and support, it helps individuals develop the knowledge, skills, and confidence they need to navigate the complexities of chronic disease management and make informed decisions about their health.

While most healthcare professionals are aware of the benefits of appropriate health education, there are several challenges and barriers that may impede its delivery (see Box I.2). Addressing these obstacles requires concerted efforts at multiple levels, including healthcare policy changes, investments in resources and infrastructure, provider training and education, and integration of technology into healthcare delivery systems. By overcoming these challenges, healthcare providers can better meet the individualized needs of patients and improve health outcomes.

Box I.2 Challenges Limiting the Impact of Health Education in Healthcare Settings

Time constraints: Healthcare providers often have limited time during patient visits to address all aspects of a patient's health, including providing personalized education. With competing demands and busy schedules, it can be challenging to allocate sufficient time for individualized education.

Limited resources: Healthcare systems may lack the resources, such as educational materials, tools, and personnel, needed to deliver personalized health education effectively. This can hinder the ability of providers to tailor educational content to the specific needs and preferences of each patient.

Training and skills: Not all healthcare providers have received adequate training or possess the necessary skills to deliver personalized health education. Effective communication, health literacy, and culturally responsive practices are essential for tailoring education to individual patients effectively.

Technological barriers: While technology has the potential to facilitate personalized health education through digital platforms, patient portals, and mobile apps, not all healthcare providers have access to or are proficient in using these tools. Additionally, patients may vary in their access to technology and digital literacy skills.

Reimbursement models: In some healthcare systems, reimbursement models may not incentivize or prioritize the delivery of personalized health education. Providers may focus more on diagnostic and treatment services than preventive or educational interventions.

Systemic challenges: Healthcare systems may face broader systemic challenges, such as fragmented care delivery, communication gaps between providers, and limited coordination across healthcare settings. These systemic issues can impede the seamless delivery of personalized health education.

Nurses, however, are in a unique position to provide more tailored health education to patients for several reasons. As the most trusted healthcare professionals for the 22nd year in a row (Brenan & Jones, 2024), nurses are trained in the principles of patient-centered care, which emphasizes collaboration, respect for patient preferences, and individualized care planning. By involving patients in the educational process and tailoring information to their specific needs and goals, nurses promote active participation and engagement in health and wellness endeavors. Nurses are also trained to take a holistic approach to patient care, considering not only the physical aspects of health but also the emotional, social, and cultural factors that influence well-being. This holistic perspective allows nurses to tailor health education to the individual needs and preferences of each patient.

Nurses often have more frequent and prolonged interactions with patients compared with other healthcare providers. This continuity of care enables nurses to develop trusting relationships with patients over time, making them well positioned to deliver personalized education and support. Effective communication is another integral cornerstone of nursing practice. Nurses are skilled at communicating complex medical information clearly, understandably, and in a culturally sensitive manner. This communication expertise allows them to personalize health education to meet the literacy levels, language preferences, and cultural backgrounds of diverse patient populations. Above all, nurses serve as advocates for their patients, ensuring that their voices are heard and their needs are met within the healthcare system. This advocacy role extends to health education, in which nurses can empower patients to make informed decisions about their health and navigate the complexities of the healthcare system.

Nurses continue to play a crucial role in health promotion, disease prevention, and the promotion of health equity. Many are involved in community-based healthcare settings, such as community health centers, public health clinics, schools, and home healthcare agencies. This allows nurses to reach underserved populations, address health disparities, and deliver culturally responsive health education tailored to the needs of local communities. Through health education, nurses can empower patients to adopt healthy lifestyle behaviors, manage chronic conditions effectively, and prevent complications through early detection and intervention. Overall, nurses' unique combination of clinical expertise, communication skills, patient advocacy, and commitment to holistic care make them invaluable providers of personalized health education to patients across diverse healthcare settings.

Chapter 1

Understanding Behavior Change

Objectives

1. Enhance healthcare professionals' understanding of factors that influence health behaviors.
2. Review behavior change intervention strategies that facilitate behavior change and promote positive outcomes.
3. Discuss the behavior change theory model.

Key Terms

- **Transtheoretical Model**
- **Stages of Change Model**
- **Motivational interviewing**
- **Health literacy assessments**
- **Plain language communication**

Behavior change refers to the process by which individuals modify their actions, habits, or attitudes in response to internal or external stimuli. It involves a series of stages through which individuals progress as they move from being unaware of a behavior and its consequences to adopting and maintaining the desired behavior over time. Effective behavior change interventions often incorporate strategies such as goal setting, self-monitoring, social support, reinforcement, environmental modification, and cognitive behavioral techniques to facilitate sustained behavior change and promote positive outcomes. Several theories and models of behavior change have been developed to understand the factors influencing individual behavior change and guide interventions aimed at promoting health and well-being. These theories include the transtheoretical model (stages of change model), social cognitive theory, health belief model, theory of planned behavior, and self-determination theory, among others.

Changing behavior can be challenging for several reasons. Many behaviors are deeply ingrained habits that have been developed over time through repetition and reinforcement. Breaking these habits and adopting new ones requires conscious effort, motivation, and persistence. People considering making changes often must confront emotional barriers, such as fear, anxiety, self-doubt, and ambivalence. Negative emotions, cognitive biases, and irrational beliefs can undermine motivation and hinder progress toward behavior change goals. Social influences such as societal norms, peer pressure, and cultural expectations can exert powerful influences on individual behavior as well. Social support and encouragement from others can facilitate behavior change, but social pressures to conform to existing norms or maintain unhealthy habits may also present obstacles. Lastly, often-overlooked influences are environmental cues and contextual factors in shaping behaviors. Physical surroundings, access to resources, socioeconomic conditions, and built environments can either facilitate or inhibit behavior change efforts.

Behavior change is rarely a simple linear process. Many behaviors are interconnected, and modifying one behavior may have ripple effects on others. Additionally, behaviors are influenced by a complex interplay of biological, psychological, social, and environmental factors, making behavior change interventions inherently multifaceted and dynamic. Sustaining motivation and willpower over time can be challenging, especially when one is faced with setbacks, temptations, or competing priorities. Motivation fluctuates over time and may be influenced by factors such as mood, stress, fatigue, and external rewards or incentives. Also important to consider is that people vary widely in their readiness for change, personality traits, learning styles, and personal preferences. What works for one individual may not be effective for another, necessitating personalized approaches tailored to individual needs, strengths, and barriers.

Addressing these challenges requires a comprehensive understanding of the factors influencing behavior change as well as the development and implementation of evidence-based strategies and interventions tailored to individual needs and contexts. By recognizing the complexity of behavior change and providing support, resources, and encouragement, individuals can enhance their likelihood of success in adopting and sustaining healthy behaviors over time.

The **transtheoretical model (TTM)** of behavior change, also known as the ***stages of change model***, was developed by psychologists James Prochaska and Carlo DiClemente in the late 1970s and early 1980s. The model provides a framework for understanding how individuals progress through distinct stages of change when modifying behavior, and it evolved through studies examining the experiences of smokers who quit on their own with those requiring further treatment to understand why some people were capable of quitting on their own. It was determined that people quit smoking if they were ready to do so. Thus, TTM focuses on the decision-making of the individual and is a model of intentional change (Prochaska & Velicer, 1997). The TTM operates on the assumption that people do not change behaviors quickly and decisively. Rather, change in behavior, especially habitual behavior, occurs continuously through a cyclical process. TTM also acknowledges that behavior change is a dynamic process that unfolds over time and involves multiple stages, each characterized by unique cognitive, emotional, and behavioral features (see Image 1.1 and Box 1.1 for a description of each stage).

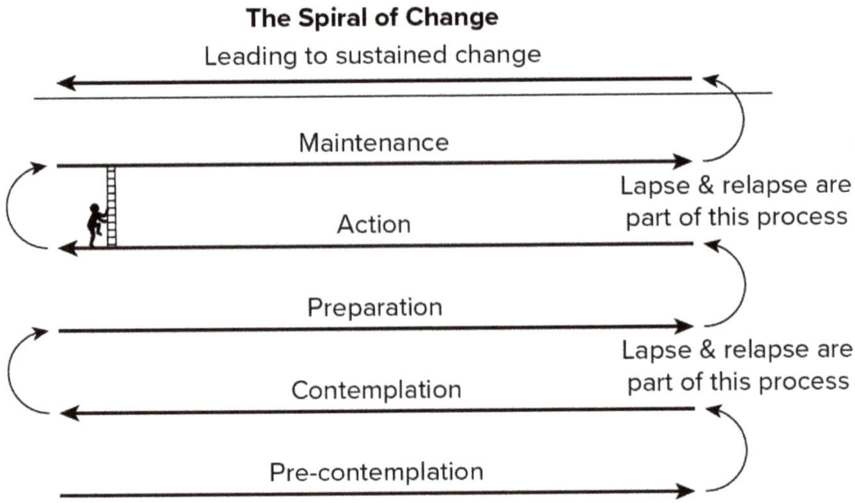

Image 1.1

Box 1.1 Distinct Stages of Change Accompanied by Examples

Precontemplation: In this stage, individuals are not yet considering behavior change and may be unaware of the need to change. They may exhibit resistance or denial regarding their behavior and its consequences.

Examples: A smoker who has not thought about quitting; someone who does not see their sedentary lifestyle as a problem.

Contemplation: During the contemplation stage, individuals become aware of the need for change and start to weigh the pros and cons of changing their behavior. They may experience ambivalence and uncertainty about whether or how to proceed with behavior change.

Examples: A smoker who acknowledges the health risks of smoking but is unsure about quitting; someone who is considering starting an exercise program but has not committed to a gym membership.

Planning/preparation: In the preparation stage, individuals are committed to changing their behavior and begin taking concrete steps toward action. They may gather information, set goals, and develop plans for initiating change within the near future.

Examples: A smoker researching resources to quit smoking; someone buying running shoes in preparation for starting an exercise routine.

Action: The action stage involves actively modifying behavior, habits, or routines in accordance with the individual's goals and action plan. This stage requires sustained effort, commitment, and perseverance to overcome challenges and maintain progress.

Examples: A smoker who has successfully quit smoking; someone who regularly attends exercise classes.

Maintenance: Once the desired behavior has been adopted, the maintenance stage focuses on sustaining the behavior change over the long term. Individuals work to prevent relapse and integrate the new behavior into their daily life, often relying on strategies such as self-monitoring, social support, and coping skills.

Examples: A former smoker who has remained smoke-free for several months; someone consistently engaging in regular physical activity.

In some versions of the model, termination is considered the final stage, in which the behavior change becomes fully ingrained and automatic. Individuals in this stage no longer experience urges to engage in the old behavior and have complete confidence in their ability to maintain the change. An example might be a former smoker who no longer has cravings for cigarettes or someone who has maintained a healthy diet and exercise routine for years without effort. However, not all behaviors may reach this stage, and relapse remains a possibility even after prolonged maintenance.

Relapse is common during any and all behavior change efforts, and maintaining long-term behavior change can be particularly challenging. Relapse can occur at any stage of change, as individuals may revert to old habits in response to stress, social triggers, or lapses in self-control, highlighting the importance of ongoing support, monitoring, and relapse prevention strategies at all stages.

The TTM also emphasizes the importance of processes of change (see Box 1.2), which are strategies or techniques that individuals use to progress through the stages of change. These processes include activities such as increasing awareness, self-evaluation, goal-setting, problem-solving, social support, and reinforcement to help guide interventions and personalize support depending on where someone is in their journey of change. Overall, the TTM provides a valuable framework for understanding the process of behavior change and guiding interventions aimed at promoting health behavior adoption and maintenance across diverse populations and contexts.

Box 1.2 Processes of Change Used to Support Behavior Change

Cognitive (Experiential) Processes

More Common in Earlier Stages (Precontemplation, Contemplation, Preparation)

1. **Consciousness raising**
    - Increasing awareness about the behavior and its consequences (e.g., reading articles, talking with a healthcare provider)
2. **Dramatic relief**
    - Emotional experiences related to the behavior change,

such as fear, inspiration, or regret (e.g., seeing a documentary that triggers concern)

3. **Environmental reevaluation**
    - Considering how the behavior affects others and the environment (e.g., realizing how secondhand smoke affects family members)
4. **Self-reevaluation**
    - Reassessing self-image with and without the unhealthy behavior (e.g., imagining yourself as a healthy, nonsmoking person)
5. **Social liberation**
    - Noticing and using societal support for change (e.g., smoke-free public spaces, support groups, public health campaigns)

Behavioral Processes

More Common in Later Stages (Planning/Preparation, Action, Maintenance)

6. **Self-liberation**
    - Making a firm commitment to change (e.g., creating a quit plan, publicly announcing your intent)
7. **Helping relationships**
    - Using support from others to aid in change (e.g., talking with a therapist, support from family or friends)

8. **Counterconditioning**
    - Substituting healthier behaviors for the unhealthy one (e.g., going for a walk instead of smoking)
9. **Reinforcement management**
    - Rewarding positive behavior changes (e.g., treating yourself for meeting a health goal)
10. **Stimulus control**
    - Changing your environment to reduce triggers (e.g., removing junk food from the house, avoiding certain places)

Motivational Interviewing

Motivational interviewing (MI) is a counseling approach that aims to facilitate behavior change by helping individuals explore and resolve ambivalence about change. Originally developed in the context of addiction treatment (Miller & Rollnick, 2013), MI has since been widely applied across various healthcare settings to promote health behavior change, disease prevention, and adherence to medical recommendations (Fixsen et al., 2005). MI emphasizes a collaborative and nonconfrontational approach between the healthcare professional and the patient. Using MI techniques can facilitate health education by doing the following:

1. **Eliciting "change talk":** MI involves prompting change talk from patients, which refers to statements expressing motivation, commitment, and confidence in making positive changes. Healthcare professionals use open-ended questions, reflections,

and affirmations to encourage patients to articulate their reasons for change and identify their own intrinsic motivations.

2. **Resolving ambivalence:** Many individuals experience ambivalence about behavior change, meaning that they have mixed feelings or conflicting motivations regarding change. MI helps individuals explore and resolve ambivalence by examining the pros and cons of both maintaining the current behavior and making a change. Healthcare professionals help patients clarify their values and priorities to strengthen their commitment to change.
3. **Empowering autonomy:** MI respects the autonomy and self-determination of the patient, recognizing that lasting behavior change must come from within the individual. Healthcare professionals support patients in making informed decisions about their health by providing information, exploring options, and fostering a sense of ownership over the change process.
4. **Enhancing self-efficacy:** MI helps patients build confidence in their ability to make and sustain behavior change. Healthcare professionals emphasize patients' strengths, past successes, and coping strategies while also offering practical support and encouragement to bolster self-efficacy.
5. **Addressing resistance and "sustain talk":** MI acknowledges that patients may express resistance or sustain talk against change. Rather than confronting or arguing against resistance, healthcare professionals use reflective listening and empathetic responses to understand the underlying reasons for resistance and explore potential barriers to change.
6. **Facilitating action planning:** MI helps patients develop concrete action plans for behavior change that are aligned with their values, preferences, and resources. Healthcare professionals collaborate with patients to set achievable goals, identify potential obstacles, and develop strategies for overcoming challenges.

MI skills include open-ended questions (O), affirmative statements (A), reflective listening (R), and summarization (S; see Table 1.1).

Table 1.1. OARS Acronym

O	***Ask open-ended*** questions that allow patients to give more information, including their feelings, attitudes, and understanding.
A	***Encourage affirmations*** to help overcome self-sabotaging or negative thoughts.
R	***Allow reflective listening*** as a way to express ambivalence.
S	***Summarize*** to let your patient know that they are being heard.

Source: Caelan Barnhart/ImageTrend, "OARS Acronym," https://www.ems1.com/ems-products/mobile-computers/articles/5-principles-to-motivational-interviewing-C6NBkSFwDPSLcI5L/. Copyright © 2020 by ImageTrend.

The "RULE" of MI is a mnemonic device used to summarize the four key principles or guidelines for practicing MI effectively (see Table 1.2). These principles are foundational to the approach and help guide healthcare professionals in their interactions with patients. The following explain what each letter in the RULE acronym represents:

1. **R: Resist the Righting Reflex:** The first principle emphasizes the importance of avoiding the urge to immediately correct or fix the patient's behavior. *Instead of imposing solutions or giving advice, we should adopt a nonjudgmental, nonconfrontational stance and focus on empathetic listening, understanding the patient's perspective, and supporting their autonomy.*
2. **U: Understand the patient's motivations:** The second principle underscores the importance of exploring and understanding the patient's motivations, values, and goals related to behavior change. *We should elicit the patient's reasons for change, identify what is important to them, and recognize the internal and external factors driving their behavior.*
3. **L: Listen with empathy:** The third principle highlights the significance of empathetic listening in MI. *We should strive to create a supportive, nonjudgmental environment where patients feel heard,*

understood, and respected. Reflective listening, validation, and affirmation help convey empathy and build rapport with patients.

4. **E: Empower the patient:** The fourth principle emphasizes the importance of supporting the patient's autonomy, self-efficacy, and capacity for change. Healthcare professionals should collaborate with patients to explore their options, set achievable goals, and develop strategies for behavior change that are aligned with their values and preferences. *By empowering patients to make informed decisions and take ownership of their health, we can facilitate sustainable behavior change.*

In summary, the RULE of MI serves as a reminder for healthcare professionals to adopt a collaborative, empathetic, and empowering approach when engaging with patients. By resisting the righting reflex, understanding the patient's motivations, listening with empathy, and empowering the patient, we can effectively facilitate behavior change and promote positive health outcomes through MI.

Table 1.2. Motivational Interviewing

R	**RESIST telling them what to do:** Avoid telling, directing, or convincing your patient about the right path to good health.
U	**UNDERSTAND their motivation:** Seek to understand their values, needs, abilities, motivations, and potential barriers to changing behaviors.
L	**LISTEN with empathy:** Seek to understand their values, needs, abilities, motivations and potential barriers to changing behaviors.
E	**EMPOWER them:** Work with your patients to set achievable goals and to identify techniques to overcome barriers.

Source: Adapted from Worksheets Library, "Motivational Interviewing," https://worksheets.clipart-library.com/worksheet/motivational-interviewing-worksheets_43.html. Copyright © by Clipart Library.

Health Literacy Assessment

Assessing health literacy levels in the clinical arena is essential for tailoring communication and education strategies to meet the needs of patients effectively. While there are various tools available to assess health literacy for research purposes, there are no best practices to assess in the clinical space. There are multiple health literacy assessment tools available, and use would depend on the workflow of each organization. Following are several approaches commonly used to assess health literacy levels:

1. **Use of screening tools:** Various validated screening tools are available to assess health literacy levels quickly and efficiently. Examples include the Rapid Estimate of Adult Literacy in Medicine, Test of Functional Health Literacy in Adults, and Newest Vital Sign. These tools typically involve reading or comprehension tasks related to health information and may be administered verbally or in written form.
2. **Observational assessment:** Clinicians can observe patients' interactions and behaviors during clinical encounters to assess their health literacy indirectly. Observational cues such as difficulty following instructions, asking frequent questions, or showing signs of confusion may indicate lower health literacy levels.
3. **Patient preferences:** Inquire about patients' preferences for receiving health information and their comfort level with various communication formats (e.g., written materials, verbal explanations, visual aids). Patients may express preferences based on their familiarity, confidence, and understanding of different communication modalities.
4. **Review of health history forms:** Reviewing patients' health history forms or intake questionnaires can provide insights into their literacy skills. Assessing patients' ability to complete forms accurately and independently can offer clues about their literacy levels and comprehension of written information.

Throughout clinical interactions, healthcare professionals can periodically assess patients' understanding of the information provided by asking open-ended questions, summarizing key points, or encouraging patients to explain concepts in their own words. Assessing patients' ability to comprehend and apply health information can help gauge their health literacy levels. Regardless of literacy levels, we should all engage in **plain language communication**. Plain language communication is a method of presenting information that is clear, concise, and easy to understand for a wide range of audiences, regardless of their literacy level or background knowledge on the topic (National Institutes of Health, 2025). The goal of plain language communication is to ensure that information is accessible and comprehensible to the intended audience, thereby promoting better understanding, informed decision-making, and improved outcomes. Observe patients' reactions and responses to gauge their comprehension and adjust communication strategies as needed to enhance understanding (see plainlanguage.gov for resources).

We should also consider cultural and linguistic factors and how these aspects may influence patients' health literacy levels and communication preferences. Tailor communication strategies to accommodate cultural differences and language barriers effectively. When language barriers exist, collaborating with professional interpreters or language services to facilitate communication with patients who have limited English proficiency is important. Ensure that interpreters are trained in medical terminology and cultural humility to facilitate accurate and effective communication.

Summary

By using a combination of these approaches, healthcare professionals can assess patients' health literacy levels and tailor communication strategies to meet their individual needs effectively. Identifying patients with limited health literacy early on can help ensure that they receive the support and resources necessary to navigate the healthcare system and make informed decisions about their health.

The following chapters will explore each stage of change and highlight how to personalize the health education we are providing to best meet the individualized needs of the people with whom we are working. Remember that behavior change is not a linear process and people may start at any stage and fall back multiple times before sustained change occurs.

Image Credit

IMG 1.1a: Copyright © 2015 Depositphotos/shekaka.

Chapter 2

Precontemplation

In this chapter, we will review which types of characteristics you might see in a patient who is not ready to make changes. We will review the kinds of comments you might hear and how you might consider responding. Upon completion of this chapter, you should be able to identify when a patient is in precontemplation and the health education that would best match this stage.

Objectives

1. List key characteristics of someone in the precontemplation stage.
2. Explain the appropriate health education for this stage.
3. Understand the relevance of health literacy.

Key Terms

- **Lack of readiness**
- **Defensiveness**
- **Denial**
- **Empathy**
- **Support**

Scenario Description

Jeff has been a smoker for most of his adult life. He enjoys smoking and believes that it helps him manage stress. Despite his recent health issues, he doesn't think his smoking habit is problematic. During his annual checkup, his doctor expresses concern about his smoking and its impact on his health, but Jeff remains unconvinced and resistant to the idea of quitting.

Health history: Diagnosed with hypertension and experiencing occasional shortness of breath. Also has had a chronic cough for more than five years. Has smoked one pack of cigarettes per day for the past 30 years.

A. Overview: Precontemplation

Characteristics of the Stage

In the precontemplation stage, individuals are not yet considering making any changes to their behavior. They may be unaware that a problem exists or simply be resistant to the idea of change. In this stage, people may have a lack of awareness about the negative consequences of their current behavior or feel overwhelmed by the challenges associated with change. They might not see the need to alter their behavior and may not even have any intention of doing so in the foreseeable future.

Key characteristics of the precontemplation stage include:

- **Denial:** Individuals may deny that their behavior is problematic or that it could have negative consequences.
- **Defensiveness:** When confronted with the need for change, they may become defensive and avoid discussions or information related to the issue.
- **Lack of readiness:** They have no intention to change in the near future.

In this stage, individuals are often resistant to advice or interventions aimed at promoting behavior change. They may not be ready to engage in discussions about their behavior, and attempts to persuade them to change may be met with resistance. It is essential for healthcare professionals (HCPs) to approach individuals in the precontemplation stage with sensitivity and empathy. Raising awareness about the need for change and gently exploring the potential benefits of changing behavior can be helpful in eventually moving individuals to the next stage of contemplation. People in this stage may also have had previous attempts to change but have since given up, and/or they may feel totally overwhelmed by the problem and see themselves as incapable of changing. It's important to note that not everyone progresses through the stages of change linearly, and individuals may cycle back and forth between stages before reaching successful behavior change. The precontemplation stage is just the first step in the process of making positive changes in one's life.

Patient Conversations: Things You Might Hear the Patient Say

During the precontemplation stage, a person may not yet be aware of or ready to acknowledge that they have a problem or need to make a change. They may be resistant to the idea of changing their behavior or unaware of the negative consequences of their actions. The following is an example of a conversation with someone in the precontemplation stage regarding their smoking habit:

> **HCP:** You mentioned that you smoke about a pack of cigarettes a day. Tell me more about your thoughts around quitting [*example of open-ended question*].
>
> **Person in precontemplation (defensive):** My smoking? Oh, it's not that big of a deal. I've been smoking for years, and I'm doing just fine. Besides, it helps me relax.
>
> **HCP:** I understand that you've been smoking for a while [*example of reflective listening*], but have you ever thought about the long-term effects it might have on your health? It's never too early to start thinking about that.

Person in precontemplation (dismissive): Oh, come on—everyone has some bad habits. I don't see the need to make a fuss about it. I've seen people who smoke all their life and live a long time.

OR

Person in precontemplation (changing the subject/denial): Look, I appreciate your concern, but I really don't want to talk about it right now.

In this example, the person in the precontemplation stage is not yet open to considering quitting smoking. They are defensive about their habit and may not fully grasp the potential negative consequences. With the earlier example, most HCPs would discuss all the benefits to quitting and spend some of the visit time trying to convince the individual to start some form of smoking cessation. However, precontemplators are not ready to engage in this kind of conversation since many do not even realize that there is a problem with their behavior.

B. Health Education for Precontemplators

Following are some key elements of health education that may be beneficial for people in the precontemplation stage, followed by examples of what the HCP might say as a continuation of the patient-provider example that was reviewed earlier.

Fostering empathy and support: Create a supportive and nonjudgmental environment where individuals feel comfortable expressing their thoughts and concerns. Encourage empathy from educators, peers, or support groups.

> *"I hear you saying that you are not ready to quit smoking right now [example of reflective listening], and that is OK. When you are ready, there are many ways we can support you."*

Raising awareness: Provide information about the health issue or behavior in question, highlighting the potential risks and consequences associated with their current behavior. The goal is to provide the individual with information, with hopes that they might recognize the importance of making a change.

> *"I am sure you know that smoking can increase your chance of lung cancer and heart disease, in addition to other breathing problems. But it is OK to not be ready to make a change. Just know that I'm here for you whenever you're ready to talk about it or if you decide to make a change." [fostering empathy and **support**]*

Highlighting benefits: Emphasize the potential benefits of adopting healthier behaviors. This could include improved physical health, enhanced mental well-being, better quality of life, increased energy, and longevity.

> *"It is OK to not be ready to make a change" [example of reflective listening]. "Here is a handout that reviews some of the health benefits you might enjoy if you stop smoking. If you have any questions after you look through it, we can have another chat."*

Accessible resources: Provide information about available resources, such as support groups, counseling services, helplines, or community programs, that can assist the patient in their journey toward change.

> *"Stopping smoking can be very hard. If you decide to make a change, here is some information on the kinds of supports and resources that we have available."*

C. Key Processes of Change for the Precontemplation Stage

Following are the most effective psychological and cognitive strategies to support someone in this stage as well as examples:

1. **Consciousness raising**

   Goal: Increase awareness of the risks and impacts of smoking.

   - Share personalized health risks (e.g., lung cancer, heart disease).
   - Provide brochures or short videos on how smoking affects the body.
   - Encourage discussions with a doctor or health educator.

2. **Dramatic relief**

   Goal: Evoke emotional reactions that highlight the consequences of smoking.

   - Show stories or testimonials from people who have suffered smoking-related illnesses.
   - Use empathy to connect ("How would you feel if your child saw you struggle to breathe?").

3. **Environmental reevaluation**

   Goal: Help the person see how their smoking affects others.

   - Talk about secondhand smoke and its impact on children or loved ones.
   - Reflect on how quitting might improve relationships or see the patient serving as a positive role model.

4. **Social liberation**

   Goal: Increase awareness of smoke-free norms and support systems.

- Highlight community policies such as smoke-free parks, workplaces, and restaurants.
- Share stories of others who have quit successfully and how their lives have improved.

What not to focus on (yet):

- Do **not** push action plans or quit dates—**they are not ready**.
- Avoid judgment or pressure, which can lead to resistance.
- Instead, focus on **planting seeds** and **building readiness**.

D. Health Literacy and Precontemplators

When considering the relationship between the precontemplation stage and health literacy, it's important to recognize that health literacy can influence a person's readiness to change and ability to engage in healthier behaviors (Coughlin, Vernon, Hatzigeorgiou & George, 2021). Here's how health literacy relates to the precontemplation stage:

Limited health literacy hindering awareness: Individuals with limited health literacy may struggle to understand health information, including information about the risks associated with their behavior. They may not recognize the severity of their health issues or the potential benefits of changing their behavior.

Difficulty understanding health information: People in the precontemplation stage may encounter difficulties when trying to comprehend written or verbal health information, especially if it is presented in complex medical terminology or uses jargon.Limited health literacy can lead to confusion and frustration, making it less likely for individuals to consider behavior change.

Barriers to seeking information: Low health literacy can act as a barrier to seeking additional information about health issues. Individuals in the precontemplation stage may not actively search for resources to learn more about their condition or behavior.

Influence of health communication: Health communication strategies tailored to the individual's health literacy level can be more effective in reaching and engaging individuals in the precontemplation stage. Clear, plain-language materials and visual aids can help bridge the gap for those with limited health literacy.

Patient-provider communication: Effective communication between healthcare providers and patients is critical, particularly for patients in the precontemplation stage. Providers should assess a patient's health literacy level and adapt their communication accordingly, ensuring that information is presented in an understandable manner.

Empowerment through health literacy: Improving health literacy can empower individuals in the precontemplation stage by enhancing their ability to access and understand health information. This empowerment may eventually lead them to progress through the stages of behavior change as they become more informed and confident about making healthier choices.

Community and peer support: Community-based health education programs and peer support groups can play a crucial role in addressing limited health literacy and encouraging individuals to move beyond precontemplation. These programs often provide a supportive environment where individuals can learn from others who have successfully made behavior changes.

Summary

In summary, health literacy plays a significant role in influencing an individual's readiness to change their behavior, especially when they are in the precontemplation stage. Healthcare providers, educators, and public health professionals can enhance the effectiveness of their efforts by considering and addressing the health literacy needs of individuals in this stage, helping them become more aware and informed about their health choices. The objective of health education during the precontemplation stage is to gently nudge individuals toward considering change and preparing them for the next stages of behavior change. Individuals may require different amounts of time to move through the stages and initiate action toward healthier behaviors. It's essential to be patient and nonjudgmental when engaging with someone in this stage, as pushing too hard may lead them to become more resistant to change. It's important to remember that the precontemplation stage is just the first step in the process of behavior change. People in this stage are often not ready to act immediately, and that's OK. The goal of health education at this stage is to plant the seeds of contemplation and readiness for change so that individuals can progress toward the next stages of the behavior change model when they are ready.

Critical Thinking Questions When Working With Someone in the Precontemplation Stage

1. What is the patient's current level of awareness about their health issue or behavior? *Assess the patient's understanding of their condition and their knowledge about the risks associated with their behavior.*
2. What factors or beliefs might be contributing to the patient's resistance to change? *Explore the patient's attitudes, beliefs, cultural factors, and past experiences that may be influencing their reluctance to consider change.*
3. Have there been any previous attempts at behavior change? *Inquire about any prior efforts the patient has made to address their health issue. Understanding past experiences can provide insights into potential barriers.*
4. What motivates the patient in other aspects of their life? *Identify the patient's personal values, interests, and sources of motivation outside of their health. This information can help in finding leverage points for change.*
5. What are the patient's goals and aspirations? *Discuss the patient's life goals and how their current behavior aligns or conflicts with those aspirations.*
6. Are there any cultural or socioeconomic factors that need to be considered in the patient's journey toward change? *Be*

aware of cultural sensitivities and socioeconomic barriers that may impact the patient's ability to make changes.

Chapter 3

Contemplation

In this chapter, we will review what types of characteristics you might see in a patient who is contemplating or considering changes. We will review the kinds of comments you might hear and how you might consider responding. Upon completion of this chapter, you should be able to identify when a patient is in contemplation and the health education that would best match this stage.

Objectives

1. List key characteristics of someone in the contemplation stage.
2. Explain the appropriate health education for this stage.
3. Understand the relevance of health literacy.

Key Terms

- **Ambivalence**
- **Decisional balance**
- **Assessing readiness for change**

Scenario Description

Julia has been living with type 2 diabetes for the past three years. During her recent checkup, her doctor expressed concern about her rising hemoglobin A1c levels and recommended that she make lifestyle changes to better manage her diabetes. Julia feels overwhelmed and unsure about where to start. She wants to improve her health but doesn't know what steps to take or how to maintain any changes she makes.

Health history: Overweight, sedentary lifestyle, poor dietary habits

A. Overview: Contemplation

Characteristics of the Stage

In the contemplation stage, individuals are thinking about making a change, as characterized by their awareness of a problem or issue, but have not yet committed to acting. There is often a sense of **ambivalence** during the contemplation stage, as they can see reasons to change their behavior, but they are still hesitant. The contemplation stage can vary in duration. Some individuals may move relatively quickly to the preparation and action stages, while others may remain in contemplation for an extended period.

Key characteristics of the contemplation stage include the following:

- *Awareness of the problem:* Individuals in the contemplation stage are aware that a problem or issue exists. This awareness may come from personal experiences, feedback from others, or external information.
- *Ambivalence:* Pros and cons of change are weighed, and individuals may feel torn between the benefits of change and the comfort of the familiar.
- *Decisional balance:* Contemplators engage in a process where they weigh the perceived benefits of change against the costs and challenges. This internal evaluation influences their readiness to move forward into the next stage of action.
- *Not yet committed to action:* The key characteristic of the contemplation stage is that individuals have not yet committed to taking specific action. They are still in the process of considering the possibility of change.

Individuals in this stage are actively considering the possibility of making a change in their behavior. They may seek information, weigh the potential benefits and challenges, and explore different strategies for change. Individuals in the contemplation stage are likely to identify potential barriers to change, such as fear of failure, concerns about the difficulty of change, or external obstacles that may impede their likelihood to change. Contemplators are open to exploring various approaches to change. This could involve seeking advice from others who have successfully made similar changes or reflecting on personal strengths and resources.

During the contemplation stage, interventions and support should focus on helping individuals resolve their ambivalence, explore motivations for change, and enhance self-efficacy. Motivational interviewing techniques can be effective during this stage to facilitate the decision-making process and move individuals closer to the action stage of behavior change. In working with contemplators, the challenge for healthcare professionals (HCPs) is to not overwhelm the patient with too much information. We should try to draw on the person's self-identified strengths and facilitate how the patient can use those skills to maintain behavior change. The content of health education should be personally relevant to the individual.

Patient Conversations: Things You Might Hear the Patient Say

During the contemplation stage, individuals are considering making a change but haven't committed to specific actions yet. People may feel conflicted about whether to make a change or continue with their current behavior. Supporting a patient in the contemplation stage requires a sensitive and understanding approach. During this stage, HCPs should be emphasizing the benefits of change instead of trying to arouse fear. Focusing on the benefits of change can create incentives for a contemplator. Following is an example of a conversation with someone in the contemplation stage regarding their management of their diabetes:

HCP: I have noticed over the past few visits that your blood sugars have been pretty high. I would like to talk with you about that.

Patient in contemplation: I check them at home and have also noticed them going up [*awareness of the problem*]. I am taking my medicine, but I have not been watching what I am eating. [*Ambivalence*] I know that I need to do better, but life has been so busy lately, and I haven't been feeling that great either.

HCP: I understand how challenging it can be to think about our food choices when we have a lot going on [*reflective listening*], but in the past, you were able to have good control of your blood sugar levels [*example of affirmation*]. Tell me what kinds of things you were doing then for better control [*example of open-ended question that focuses on identifying patient's strengths*].

Patient in contemplation: Well, when I was first diagnosed with diabetes, I was married, and my kids were at home. They really helped me to meal prep. Now I am divorced, and the kids are away in college. I spend a lot more time alone and don't really feel like cooking for just myself, so I eat out more with friends, and I also drink wine a lot more now than I did before. I know that doesn't help because alcohol is just like sugar [*awareness of the problem*]. That is an area where I need to cut back, but I am so stressed out most of the time that I really like to relax with a glass of wine at night. There is a lot to consider.

In this example, the person in the contemplation stage recognizes that there are changes that she can make to improve her blood sugar levels. However, she has not committed to any one thing. With this example, most HCPs might try to scare the patient into making changes by telling her that uncontrolled blood sugars over time can lead to permanent kidney damage and eventual dialysis. However, contemplators would benefit more from discussing benefits to change and how to work through the perceived barriers. Working through a pros and cons list together may help the HCP better understand the challenges or fears that the individual is working through (see Image 3.1, pro/con decisional balance matrix) and will help assess readiness for change. Fear-arousal messages (i.e., scare tactics) generally should be avoided because they serve to undermine self-efficacy and can dampen optimism about the prospects for change.

	Not Changing Behavior	Changing Behavior
Pros	**Box 1**: What is something good that could come from *not* taking this action?	**Box 4**: What is something good that could come from taking this action?
Cons	**Box 2**: What is something bad that could come from *not* taking this action?	**Box 3**: What is something bad that could come from taking this action?

Image 3.1

B. Health Education for Contemplators

Following are some key elements of health education that may be beneficial for people in the contemplation stage as well as examples of what the HCP might say as a continuation of the patient-provider example that was reviewed earlier.

Explore ambivalence: Acknowledge and explore the patient's ambivalence about making a change. Help them articulate both the reasons for considering a change and the barriers or concerns they may have.

"If you do make a change, what are you most afraid of?"

"Let's explore the pros/cons of changing this behavior."

Provide information: Offer balanced and accurate information about the potential benefits of change and the risks of maintaining the current behavior. Help the patient make an informed decision.

"Better control of your blood sugar will help you feel better, more energetic and less stressed out. Over time, better control will also help protect your kidneys, heart, and circulation."

Highlight personal motivations: Explore the patient's personal motivations for change. What benefits do they foresee? How does the current behavior impact their life? Helping the patient connect emotionally to their reasons for change can enhance motivation.

"How do you think your life might change if your diabetes were better controlled?"

"Currently, how does your diabetes interfere with what you want to do with your life?"

Discuss previous attempts: Inquire about the patient's past attempts to make similar changes. Understanding previous successes and challenges can provide insights into effective strategies for the future.

"The last time you tried to make some changes, what challenges did you run into?"

"If you were to make a change, what kind of support do you think you might need?"

Assess readiness for change: Assess the patient's readiness for change without pressuring them. Ask open-ended questions about their willingness to take small steps toward change and gauge their level of commitment.

> *"On a scale of 1 to 10, where 1 is no confidence and 10 is the most confidence, how ready do you feel you are to make some changes related to your diabetes?"*

> *"What kinds of small changes do you think you might be willing to make?"*

Enhance self-efficacy: Support the patient in building confidence and self-efficacy by emphasizing their strengths and past successes. Encourage them to recognize their ability to make positive changes.

> *"Your hemoglobin A1c was at goal in the past, which means that you were able to do what you need to keep your sugar controlled."*

> *"You have already identified a few areas where you can make some small changes that would help your numbers."*

C. Key Processes of Change for the Contemplation Stage

The following cognitive and emotional strategies can help the individual resolve ambivalence and build motivation to take action; also included are examples:

1. **Consciousness raising**

   Goal: Provide information about diabetes and its consequences to increase awareness.

   - Explain how uncontrolled diabetes leads to complications such as kidney failure, nerve damage, or vision loss.

- Offer resources on the benefits of lifestyle changes and early intervention.

2. **Self-reevaluation**

   Goal: Help the person assess how their current behavior aligns with their values and self-image.

   - Reflect on questions such as *"How do you see yourself in five years if nothing changes?"*
   - Encourage journaling or talking about how they want to feel and live.

3. **Environmental reevaluation**

   Goal: Help them understand how their health behaviors affect others.

   - Discuss how managing diabetes can allow them to be more present for family or avoid burdening loved ones later.
   - Explore how their role as a parent, grandparent, or caregiver is affected by their health.

4. **Dramatic relief**

   Goal: Elicit emotional responses to the seriousness of their condition or the hope of change.

   - Watch a video or read a story about someone who struggled but eventually managed their diabetes well.
   - Discuss fears the patient may have about their health and offer supportive validation.

5. **Social liberation**

   Goal: Highlight available options and supports for healthier living.

- Introduce community diabetes programs, dietitian services, or peer support groups.
- Normalize help-seeking and show that resources are accessible and stigma-free.

What to avoid:

- Don't push the person into action before they're ready.
- Avoid scare tactics—use **balanced information** and **empathy**.

D. Health Literacy and Contemplators

When considering the relationship between the contemplation stage and health literacy, it's important to recognize that health literacy can influence a person's understanding of need for change, their readiness to change, and their ability to engage in new behaviors. Here's how health literacy relates to the contemplation stage:

Understanding health information: In the contemplation stage, individuals are actively seeking information and considering making changes to their health behavior. Adequate health literacy ensures that they can understand the information presented to them, including the potential benefits and risks of behavior change. People in the contemplation stage may struggle to comprehend complex health information or misinterpret the information they receive. This can lead to confusion, uncertainty, and indecision about whether or how to change their behavior.

Difficulty weighing options: Contemplating behavior change involves weighing the pros and cons of changing versus maintaining the status quo. Individuals with limited health literacy may struggle to evaluate the information and options available to them, making it challenging to make informed decisions about behavior change.

Lack of knowledge about available resources and difficulty navigating resources: People in the contemplation stage may be unaware of the resources, support services, or treatment options available to help them make behavior changes. Limited health literacy can prevent individuals from accessing or using these resources effectively.

Ineffective communication with HCPs: Effective communication between patients and HCPsis essential for facilitating behavior change. Individuals with limited health literacy may have difficulty understanding medical terminology, following instructions, or asking questions during healthcare encounters, which can impede the exchange of information and shared decision-making.

Overreliance on misinformation or personal beliefs: In the absence of accurate health information, individuals in the contemplation stage may rely on misinformation, myths, or personal beliefs to guide their decision-making about behavior change. This can lead to suboptimal health outcomes if the information is inaccurate or contradicts evidence-based guidelines.

Cultural and linguistic barriers: Cultural and linguistic factors can also influence health literacy and impact an individual's ability to contemplate behavior change. Language barriers, cultural beliefs, and communication preferences may affect how individuals perceive health information and engage with HCPs.

To address health literacy during the contemplation stage, HCPs and educators can employ the following strategies:

- *Clear and accessible information:* Provide health information in clear, plain language that is easy to understand. Use visuals, diagrams, and multimedia tools to enhance comprehension.
- *Interactive education:* Engage individuals in interactive educational activities that promote active learning and understanding.
- *Supportive communication:* Encourage open communication with HCPs. Ensure that patients feel comfortable asking questions and seeking clarification.
- *Cultural humility:* Tailor health information to be culturally sensitive and relevant to the individual's background. This enhances understanding and resonates with diverse populations.

Summary

In summary, addressing health literacy concerns in the contemplation stage requires a multifaceted approach that involves providing clear, understandable health information; promoting effective communication; addressing cultural and linguistic barriers; and supporting patients in accessing and using available resources. Health literacy empowers individuals to make informed decisions about their health. This includes understanding the consequences of maintaining the current behavior and potential benefits of making a change. Using a decisional balance matrix may help to understand ambivalence. The objective of health education during the contemplation stage is to support individuals in exploring their motivations, values, concerns, and assess readiness for behavior change. The health education should aim to provide individuals with the information, resources, and support they need to make informed decisions about their health as they consider the possibility of behavior change.

Always respect the patient's autonomy and readiness to change. Avoid pushing them into action before they feel ready. Recognize that everyone progresses at their own pace. Remember that scare tactics can negatively affect self-efficacy and decrease the likelihood of change. Our main role is to help the patient work through their ambivalence and provide them with information that will assist them to make informed decisions that will hopefully propel them into the next stage of change: planning/preparation.

Consider using motivational interviewing techniques, which involve guiding the patient toward recognizing and resolving their ambivalence. This approach helps elicit the patient's intrinsic motivation for change. Establish trust and rapport with the patient. A trusting relationship provides a safe space for the patient to discuss their thoughts and concerns about making a change. Practice active listening to understand the patient's perspective. Allow them to express their ambivalence, concerns, and motivations for change without judgment. Engaging in critical thinking questions can help individuals in the contemplation stage explore their motivations, assess potential barriers, and gain a deeper understanding of the change they are considering. Following are some critical thinking questions that can be helpful during this stage. These questions are designed to prompt reflection and encourage individuals in the contemplation stage to think critically about their readiness for change, motivations, and potential strategies for moving forward. It's important to approach these discussions with empathy, allowing the individual to explore their thoughts and feelings without judgment.

Critical Thinking Questions When Working With Someone in the Contemplation Stage

1. Motivation for change: *What are the main reasons you're considering making this change in your life? How would your life be different if you decided to make this change?*
2. Pros and cons: *What do you see as the potential benefits of making this change? Can you identify any potential challenges or drawbacks to making this change?*
3. Past experiences: *Have you tried to make a similar change in the past? If so, what worked well, and what didn't? How might your past experiences influence your approach to making this change now?*
4. Knowledge and information: *What information or resources have you sought out to better understand the change you're thinking about? Are there specific aspects of the change that you feel you need more information about?*
5. Internal and external motivations: *How much of your motivation to change comes from within, and how much is influenced by external factors? What values or personal goals align with the change you want to make?*

6. Readiness for change: *On a scale from 1 to 10, how ready do you feel to make this change right now? What would it take to move that number higher?*
7. Support system: *Who in your life might be supportive of this change? How can they help you during this process? Are there potential sources of negativity or resistance to change in your social circles?*
8. Understanding of the change process: *How do you envision the process of making this change unfolding over time? What small steps do you think you could take to move closer to making this change a reality?*
9. Self-reflection: *What strengths or skills do you possess that could help you in the process of making this change? How do you typically respond to challenges or setbacks, and how might this impact your ability to make this change?*
10. Barriers and solutions: *What obstacles or barriers do you anticipate in making this change? How might you overcome them? Are there potential roadblocks that you haven't yet considered?*

Image Credit

IMG 3.1: Adapted from Agency for Healthcare Research and Quality, "Decisional Balance Worksheet," https://www.ahrq.gov/ncepcr/tools/obesity-kit/obtoolkit-tool14.html, U.S. Department of Health and Human Services, 2014.

Chapter 4

Planning/Preparation

In this chapter, we will review which types of characteristics you might see in a patient who has decided to make a change. We will review the kinds of comments you might hear and how you might consider responding. Upon completion of this chapter, you should be able to identify when a patient is in the planning/preparation stage and the health education that would best match their needs.

Objectives

1. List key characteristics of someone in the planning/preparation stage.
2. Explain the appropriate health education for this stage.
3. Understand the relevance of health literacy.

Key Terms

- **Support**
- **Action plan**
- **Resources**
- **SMART goals**

Scenario Description

Sarah (age 35) has recently been informed by her doctor that she is prediabetic and needs to lose weight to avoid developing type 2 diabetes.

She is motivated to make changes and has started researching weight loss strategies. She has made some small changes, such as drinking more water and reducing her soda intake, but is looking for a more structured weight loss plan to follow.

Health status: Overweight, with a body mass index of 33, and prediabetes (hemoglobin A1c = 6.1%). Sedentary job, irregular exercise habits.

A. Overview: Planning/Preparation

Characteristics of the Stage

The preparation/planning stage is a crucial phase in the transtheoretical model. In the preparation/planning stage, individuals have made a decision to change their behavior and are actively getting ready to take action within the next 30 days. The individual has decided to change their behavior and begun to think about how to do so. While individuals in the preparation stage have not yet taken definitive action to change their behavior, they may begin to implement small changes or experiment to test out new behaviors and build momentum toward larger changes. Individuals in the preparation stage work to build confidence in their ability to make and sustain behavior change. They may draw on past successes or seek encouragement from others to bolster their self-efficacy. Individuals may seek **support** from friends, family members, or support groups to help them stay motivated and accountable during the change process. They may share their goals and **action plans** with others and enlist their support in achieving them.

Key characteristics of the planning/preparation stage include:

- *Increased commitment:* Individuals in the preparation stage have decided to change their behavior and are committed to taking action. They have recognized the importance of making a change and are motivated to move forward with their plans.
- *Concrete action plans:* People in the preparation stage are engaged in developing specific action plans for behavior change. They may

identify goals, set deadlines, and outline the steps they need to take to initiate change.

- *Gathering information and resources:* Individuals actively seek out information, resources, and support services that can assist them in making behavior changes. They may research treatment options, consult with healthcare providers (HCPs), or seek guidance from trusted sources.
- *Identifying barriers and solutions:* People in the preparation stage anticipate potential obstacles or challenges to behavior change and develop strategies for overcoming them. They may identify triggers, high-risk situations, or internal barriers that could hinder progress and brainstorm ways to address these challenges.
- *Setting realistic goals:* People in the preparation stage set realistic, achievable goals for behavior change that are consistent with their values, preferences, and capabilities. They may break larger goals into smaller, more manageable steps to increase the likelihood of success.

An **action plan** is a detailed outline or strategy that lists specific steps and tasks individuals will take to achieve their goals. In the context of behavior change, an action plan is a roadmap that helps individuals move from intention to action by breaking down their goals into manageable, actionable steps. Following are the key components of an action plan:

- Goal statement: Clearly define the desired outcome or behavior change goal.
- Specific actions: Identify the actions or behaviors that individuals will take to work toward their goal. These actions should be concrete, observable behaviors that move individuals closer to their desired outcome.
- Timeline: Establish a timeline for completing each action or task. Determine when each action will be initiated and completed and set deadlines for achieving milestones along the way.

- Resources needed: Identify any resources, tools, or support services that individuals will need to implement their action plan successfully. This may include access to information, financial resources, social support, or professional assistance.
- Barriers and solutions: Anticipate potential obstacles, challenges, or barriers that may arise during the implementation of the action plan. Develop strategies and solutions for overcoming these barriers and staying on track toward the goal.
- Monitoring and evaluation: Determine how progress toward the goal will be monitored and evaluated. Define specific criteria or indicators for measuring success and establish a process for tracking progress, adjusting strategies, and reviewing outcomes.

Identify individuals or support systems that can provide accountability, encouragement, and assistance throughout the implementation of the action plan. This may include friends, family members, HCPs, or support groups. Recognize that action plans may need to be adjusted or modified based on changing circumstances, feedback, or new information. Maintain flexibility and openness to revising the action plan as needed to ensure continued progress toward the goal.

During the preparation stage, interventions and support should focus on helping individuals access the resources they will need to make the change and increase their self-confidence (see Image 4.1). This self-efficacy is crucial for maintaining motivation and perseverance during challenging times. During this stage, individuals have acknowledged the importance of changing their behavior and are committed to doing so. They have recognized the need for change and are mentally prepared to act. Individuals in this stage are laying the groundwork for behavior change and are poised to move forward with their plans. Helping people in this stage set **s**pecific, **m**easurable, **a**chievable, **r**elevant, and **t**ime-bound (SMART) goals will facilitate measuring progress during the behavior change process.

A **SMART goal** is a **s**pecific, **m**easurable, **a**chievable, **r**elevant, and **t**ime-bound goal that provides a clear and structured framework for setting and achieving objectives (see Box 4.1 for examples). *SMART* is an acronym that breaks down the key components of effective goal setting.

Specific: A specific goal clearly defines what is to be achieved. It answers the questions "What do I want to accomplish?" "Why is it important?" "Who is involved?" "Where will it happen?" "What are the requirements and constraints?"

Measurable: A measurable goal includes criteria for tracking progress and determining when the goal has been achieved. It answers the questions "How much?" "How many?" "How will I know when it is accomplished?"

Achievable: An achievable goal is realistic and attainable within the resources, constraints, and timeframe available. It considers factors such as skills, knowledge, resources, and support needed to achieve the goal.

Relevant: A relevant goal aligns with broader objectives, values, and priorities. It is meaningful and contributes to personal or organizational growth, improvement, or success.

Time-bound: A time-bound goal specifies a target date or deadline for achieving the goal. It creates a sense of urgency and helps maintain focus and motivation. It answers the question "When will it be accomplished?"

Box 4.1 Examples of SMART goals

The following examples of **SMART** goals provide clear and specific targets for improving health outcomes, making them actionable and achievable within a defined time frame:

Weight loss goal:

Specific: Lose 10 pounds in three months.

Measurable: Track weight weekly using a scale.

Achievable: Aim for a gradual weight loss of 1 to 2 pounds per week through a combination of healthy eating and regular exercise.

Relevant: Improve overall health and reduce the risk of obesity-related health conditions.

Time-bound: Achieve the goal within three months.

Physical activity goal:

Specific: Run a 5K race within three months.

Measurable: Track progress by recording weekly running distances and times.

Achievable: Follow a training plan designed for beginners, gradually increasing running distance and intensity.

Relevant: Improve cardiovascular fitness, endurance, and mental well-being.

Time-bound: Complete a 5K race within three months.

Nutrition goal:

Specific: Eat five servings of fruits and vegetables daily for three months.

Measurable: Keep a food diary to track daily fruit and vegetable intake.

Achievable: Plan meals and snacks to include a variety of fruits and vegetables throughout the day.

Relevant: Increase intake of essential vitamins, minerals, and fiber to support overall health and well-being.

Time-bound: Consistently meet the goal of consuming five servings of fruits and vegetables daily for three months.

In the next section is an example of a conversation with someone in the preparation stage regarding their management of their weight.

Patient Conversations: Things You Might Hear the Patient Say

As individuals are actively planning and preparing to take action to modify their behavior within the near future, it is important for HCPs to acknowledge their efforts and willingness to act and affirm their decision to make positive changes to their health behaviors.

Patient in preparation: I know that you have been telling me for a while that I need to lose weight, so I decided I am going to make some changes.

HCP: That is fantastic [*positive affirmation*]! Tell me a bit more about what you have decided to do [*open-ended question to explore readiness*].

Patient in preparation: Well, I have cleaned out my pantry and gotten rid of all the junk food, so I won't be tempted to snack on unhealthy stuff. And I have been researching different gyms and thinking about which one would be the best fit for me.

HCP: Making healthier food choices and doing exercise are two great ways to meet your weight loss goals [*example of summarizing*]. What kinds of things are you considering for the gym?

Patient in preparation: Cost is a big factor and so is whether they offer group classes. I think the classes might help me in the beginning.

In this example, the patient has been thinking about ways to meet their weight loss goals. These statements reflect a readiness to change and some active planning. They have decided to throw away foods that might be problematic but have yet to commit to exercise or even the purchasing of healthier foods. This is a crucial juncture, in which the right or wrong kind of support could push the patient in either direction. Paying attention to the patient's priorities and offering guidance and support without imposing your own agenda or values is paramount.

B. Health Education for Planners

Following are some key elements of health education that may be beneficial for people in the planning/preparation stage as well as examples of what an HCP might say as a continuation of the patient-provider example that was reviewed earlier.

Acknowledge and validate their readiness: Recognize and validate the patient's commitment to change. Acknowledge their efforts and willingness to act and affirm their decision to make positive changes to their health behaviors.

"I think it is great that you are thinking about ways to help you to meet your weight loss goals."

"I am so excited to hear that you are ready to make some changes."

Provide information and education: Offer tailored information, resources, and education to support the patient's preparation efforts.

Provide evidence-based information about the benefits of behavior change, available treatment options, and strategies for overcoming barriers to change.

> *"I understand your concerns about costs. Here is a list of gyms that offer discounts with certain health insurances. This might save you some money."*

> *"I can give you a referral to a nutritionist to help you learn how to find alternatives to the junk food that you just threw away."*

Assist in goal setting: Help the patient set realistic, achievable goals for behavior change. Collaboratively identify SMART goals that align with the patient's values, preferences, and capabilities.

> *"Since you sound like you are ready to make some changes, I think setting a small goal for you to work on before our next visit might help. What is something that you would want to work on between now and our next visit?"*

Offer practical strategies and tools: Provide practical strategies, tools, and techniques to help the patient prepare for behavior change. Offer guidance on how to develop action plans, identify potential obstacles, and develop coping strategies for managing challenges.

> *"I want you to think about those foods that you don't want to eat and what you might want to replace them with. Then make a list and leave this on your fridge as a reminder when you might be struggling."*

> *"Meal prepping can be very useful. Would you like to talk about how that might work?"*

Encourage self-efficacy: Foster the patient's belief in their ability to make and sustain behavior change. Offer encouragement, positive reinforcement, and support to help build the patient's confidence and self-efficacy.

> "I remember that the last time you started going to the gym, you immediately started feeling like you had more energy."
>
> "On a scale of 0 to 10 [*use confidence ruler; see below*], how confident are you that you will join a gym within the next month?" [*If their confidence is less than 7, than reassess goal or talk about what might increase their confidence.]*

On a scale of 0 to 10, how IMPORTANT is it for you right now to change?

0___1___2___3___4___5___6___7___8___9___10

Not at all Important — Extremely Important

On a scale of 0 to 10, how CONFIDENT are you that you could make this change?

0___1___2___3___4___5___6___7___8___9___10

Not at all Confident — Extremely Confident

Image 4.1

C. Key Processes of Change for the Preparation Stage

The following strategies help people develop a clear plan, build confidence, and remove barriers to action.

1. **Self-liberation**

   Goal: Strengthen belief in their ability to change and commit to a plan.

   - Encourage verbal or written commitment: *"I'm going to start walking 20 minutes each morning."*
   - Help them set **SMART goals.**
   - Support statements such as "I can do this," "This time is different," or "I'm ready."

2. **Helping relationships**

   Goal: Build a support system to encourage follow-through.

   - Encourage them to tell a friend or family member about their plan.
   - Suggest joining a diabetes prevention group or fitness class or meeting with a dietitian.
   - Ask, "*Who can help you stay motivated or walk with you?*"

3. **Social liberation**

   Goal: Increase awareness of available resources and support.

   - Share community programs, meal planning apps, or culturally relevant nutrition tools.
   - Let them know they are not alone—others are doing this, too.

4. **Stimulus control**

   Goal: Help them shape their environment to support the upcoming behavior change.

   - Plan to remove junk food from the home.
   - Place walking shoes near the door as a visual cue.
   - Set phone reminders for meals or workouts.

D. Health Literacy and Preparation/Planners

When working with individuals in the preparation stage of behavior change, it's important to consider their health literacy level to ensure that they have the knowledge, skills, and understanding necessary to effectively prepare for behavior change. Following are some important considerations related to health literacy for individuals in the preparation stage:

Tailor information: Provide information and education that is tailored to the individual's health literacy level, preferences, and needs. Use plain language, avoid jargon, and break down complex concepts into simpler, more understandable terms.

Clarify misconceptions: Address any misconceptions or misunderstandings the individual may have about their health condition, treatment options, or behavior change goals. Take the time to clarify information and answer questions to ensure accurate understanding.

Check understanding: Assess the individual's understanding of the information provided by asking open-ended questions, encouraging them to summarize key points, or requesting feedback. Be attentive to signs of confusion or uncertainty and address any gaps in understanding.

Involve support persons: Involve support persons, such as family members, caregivers, or friends, in the education and preparation process. Encourage these individuals to attend appointments, participate in discussions, and reinforce key messages at home.

HCPs and educators can employ the following strategies to address concerns with low health literacy:

- Using visual aids: Incorporate visual aids, such as diagrams, charts, or illustrations, to supplement verbal information and enhance comprehension. Visual aids can help reinforce key concepts and make information more accessible to individuals with varying levels of health literacy.
- Offering multiple formats: Present information in multiple formats to accommodate different learning styles and preferences. Offer written materials, audiovisual resources, online resources, or interactive tools to enhance engagement and accessibility.
- Providing supportive resources: Offer additional resources, such as pamphlets, handouts, websites, or community programs, that individuals can refer to for further information and support. Ensure that these resources are easy to understand and readily accessible.

Summary

In summary, this stage should focus on ensuring that the individual has the necessary knowledge to move forward with their plans. Celebrate the patient's successes, no matter how small, and acknowledge their progress toward behavior change. Offer praise, recognition, and positive reinforcement to reinforce their motivation and commitment to change. When working with someone in the planning or preparation stage of behavior change, critical thinking questions can help guide discussions and support the individual in developing actionable plans for change. By creating an action plan, individuals can clarify their goals, establish a roadmap for change, and increase their likelihood of success in achieving their desired outcomes. Action plans provide a structured framework for turning intentions into actions and moving closer towards meaningful behavior change.

Providers and educators need to ensure they have created a supportive environment that encourages individuals to ask questions, seek clarification, and express concerns. Emphasize that there are no stupid questions and that asking for help is an important part of the learning process. This is a good stage to encourage the patient to enlist the support of friends, family members, or support groups to help them stay motivated and accountable. We may have to offer guidance on how to communicate their goals and needs to others and how to seek support when necessary. By integrating cultural humility into health education during the planning phase, HCPs can promote inclusivity, respect, and effectiveness in supporting individuals from diverse cultural backgrounds in their behavior change efforts.

Respect the individual's autonomy and preferences in how they receive and process information. Allow them to take an active role in their learning process and modify educational interventions to their unique needs and preferences. By providing tailored support, guidance, and encouragement, HCPs can empower patients in the preparation stage to act toward positive behavior change and achieve their health goals. Schedule regular follow-up appointments to check in on the patient's progress, offer validation and encouragement, and address any concerns or challenges that arise. Adjust strategies as needed, especially as the patient progresses to action. As we intentionally consider these items, HCPs can ensure that individuals in the preparation stage receive the information, support, and resources they need to effectively prepare for behavior change and make informed decisions about their health. These critical thinking questions can help individuals in the planning or preparation stage of behavior change develop realistic, actionable plans for change; address potential obstacles; and build confidence in their ability to succeed. By engaging in thoughtful reflection and problem-solving, individuals can set themselves up for success as they work toward their behavior change goals.

Critical Thinking Questions When Working With Someone in the Planning/Preparation Stage

Clarifying goals and motivations

- *What specific behavior change goals are you hoping to achieve? Why are these goals important to you? What motivates you to make this change? How do these goals align with your values, priorities, and aspirations?*

Identifying strategies and resources

- *What steps have you taken so far to prepare for behavior change? What resources or support services do you anticipate needing to achieve your goals? How can you leverage your strengths, skills, and support network to help you succeed?*

Addressing potential barriers and challenges

- *What obstacles do you anticipate encountering in making this change? How have you dealt with similar challenges in the past? What strategies were effective? What additional support or resources might you need to overcome these barriers?*

Developing action plans

- *What specific actions or behaviors will you take to work toward your goals? When and where will you take these actions? How often? For how long? How will you monitor your progress and evaluate your success along the way?*

Assessing confidence and self-efficacy

- *How confident are you in your ability to make and sustain this behavior change? What past experiences or successes can you draw upon to build your confidence? What strategies can you use to boost your belief in your ability to succeed?*

Exploring social support and accountability

- *Who in your support network can provide encouragement, guidance, or accountability? How can you communicate your goals and needs to others and enlist their support? What role do you envision others playing in supporting you on your journey?*

Reflecting on personal values and meaning

- *How does making this behavior change align with your broader values and life goals? What impact do you anticipate this change will have on your overall well-being and quality of life? What deeper meaning does this change hold for you?*

Creating contingency plans

- *What will you do if you encounter setbacks or slip-ups along the way? How will you handle moments of temptation, cravings, or urges to revert to old habits? What strategies can you use to stay motivated and resilient in the face of challenges?*

Image Credit

IMG 4.1: Lark, "Confidence Ruler," https://www.lark.com/resources/how-to-use-motivational-interviewing-to-boost-motivation. Copyright © by Lark Technologies, Inc.

Chapter 5

Action

In this chapter, we will review which types of characteristics you might see in a patient who is actively involved in behavior change. We will review the kinds of comments you might hear and how you might consider responding. Upon completion of this chapter, you should be able to identify when a patient is in the action stage and the health education that would best match their needs.

Objectives

1. List key characteristics of someone in the action stage.
2. Explain the appropriate health education for this stage.
3. Understand the relevance of health literacy.

Key Terms

- **Encouragement**
- **Coping strategies**
- **Identifying triggers**
- **Goal setting**

Scenario Description

Maya is a 42-year-old elementary school teacher and mother of two. Over the past year, she's been feeling overwhelmed, anxious, and physically drained. After talking with her doctor and a therapist, she realized that chronic stress was affecting both her mental and physical health—leading to insomnia, emotional eating, and tension headaches. She is ready to make changes so that she can feel better.

Health history: Perimenopausal, slightly elevated blood pressure (138/88), does walk daily with her dog; body mass index of 30

A. Overview: Action

Characteristics of the Stage

The action phase represents a time when individuals begin to actively implement their behavior change. The change is no longer just about the intention or planning—it's about taking concrete steps toward their goal. The changes are typically short-term at first but are intended to lead to lasting habits. Action is often sustained over a period of weeks or a couple of months. Individuals start to engage in visible, noticeable actions to change their behavior. There may be fluctuations, but the person is actively focused on achieving success. They often seek or receive social support from friends, family, or professional resources during the action phase. This support helps them cope with challenges and boosts motivation. Relapse or setbacks are more likely to occur during this phase and should be considered a normal part of the change process. While some may return to old habits temporarily, this doesn't mean failure. What matters is getting back on track.

Key characteristics of the action phase include the following:

- *Changes actively being made:* Individuals have done the necessary planning to move into action. The person is doing something specific and intentional to change a behavior and change is visible (e.g. going to the gym, attending therapy, buying healthier foods).
- *Commitment and consistency:* People in the action stage are committed to their goal and working hard to maintain consistency in their new behaviors. People will often track their progress through journaling or apps. It is a time when they will also gain an

increased awareness of what works and what doesn't to sustain their change.

- *Increased self-efficacy:* As individuals engage in the desired behavior and experience successes, their self-confidence in their ability to continue the change grows. They begin to believe that they can make lasting changes.

To make the behavior change sustainable, individuals may use specific strategies or interventions such as planning, self-monitoring, behavior substitution, or setting goals. Motivation remains high in the action phase, but it may need to be reinforced regularly. Individuals often seek social support, tools, or professional guidance during this phase. They are motivated but still need **encouragement**, rewards, and reminders to stay on track. People often set small, achievable goals and track their progress to stay focused and motivated. Building new habits requires learning **coping strategies**, problem-solving, and adaptability. They may change their surroundings to support success (e.g., removing **triggers**, joining new communities). There's often a focus on day-to-day or week-to-week progress to build confidence.

Patient Conversations: Things You Might Hear the Patient Say

Patient in action: I have made some changes, and I am doing a few things to try to decrease the stress in my life.

Healthcare provider (HCP): I am so proud of you and happy to hear that [*positive affirmation*]. Tell me more about the kinds of things that you are doing [*open-ended question to allow her to give concrete examples*].

Patient in action: Well, I started incorporating daily relaxation techniques, like meditating in the mornings before work for 10 minutes and doing some deep breathing during the day if I find myself feeling tense.

HCP: Meditating is a wonderful way to decrease stress [*example of summarizing*]. Have you noticed that your headaches have decreased since you started *[educating on connecting behavior change to health outcome]?*

Patient in action: Yes! I am using less Tylenol.

HCP: I know you had mentioned that you were seeing a therapist. What other people do you have in your life to help you when you are feeling overwhelmed [*exploring use of social supports*]?

In this example, the patient has been actively making changes that will decrease the stress in her life. These statements reflect what she has prioritized and feels ready to change. She has committed to adding daily meditation and deep breathing, and the provider is trying to help her connect the dots and understand how these changes are affecting her health in a positive way. This is a way to reinforce the behavior change. The provider is also trying to ensure that she has additional resources for support, understanding that relapse is very likely during this stage.

B. Health Education for Actioners

Following are some key elements of health education that may be beneficial for people in the action stage as well as examples of what the HCP might say as a continuation of the patient-provider example that was reviewed earlier.

Coping and problem-solving strategies: Discuss how to handle setbacks, cravings, or stress associated with the change without giving up. Role-playing common triggers and appropriate responses is useful during this stage.

"I know that work is often a source of your stress. Have you considered talking with your school principal to manage some of that? What might you say when you go and speak with your boss?"

"Let's think about how you might handle a big project that gets handed to you with a quick turnaround time."

Self-monitoring tools: Review ways to use journaling, apps, or logs to track behavior and progress. Help them to recognize patterns that may lead to setbacks or success!

"You could keep a daily log of your stress levels and note any specific triggers. Let's review it next time to see how you're progressing and if we need to adjust your approach."

"You have mentioned that the beginning of the school year is a particularly stressful time for you. What kinds of strategies will you incorporate this year so that you don't feel so overwhelmed?"

Understanding the "why": Reinforce the connection between the new behavior and health outcomes. Provide updated, personalized health risk information so that they see results.

"Using less Tylenol for your headaches probably means that your blood pressure has also been more controlled. Have you seen lower numbers when you check it at home? Today your blood pressure is better than usual."

"I also see that you lost a little bit of weight since your last visit. Why do you think that is?"

Building a support system: Discuss how to seek and maintain social support (e.g., joining a group, finding a workout buddy, talking with family about the desired outcomes). This also might require modifications to their home, work, or social environment to reduce temptations or obstacles.

"Your therapist can be a great support for you during this time, but who else do you think might be a good resource for you?"

"I recently took a fantastic online breathwork class. Is this something you might be interested in?"

Relapse prevention planning: Build confidence in communication skills to ask for help or encouragement. This would also facilitate setting boundaries with people who might not support the change, which could trigger a relapse. Normalize occasional setbacks and frame them as learning opportunities.

"When anyone changes old habits, it is very common to relapse. That is the norm and not the exception. So, it is OK if you forget to meditate or if you start to feel anxious and overwhelmed. How will you ask for help if you feel yourself slipping back and feeling very stressed?"

Maintaining momentum: Emphasize **goal setting** as a motivational and organizational tool. Help them understand how to use positive reinforcement (both internal and external rewards) to stay motivated and discuss strategies to prevent burnout (e.g., variety, fun, celebrating milestones). Positive reinforcement helps to strengthen the patient's commitment to the change.

"You have been meditating for nearly two months, which is quite an accomplishment. How are you celebrating this milestone?"

"I see that you've started incorporating deep breathing exercises every day. That's a great step in reducing stress, and it's important for your overall well-being."

C. Key Processes of Change for the Action Stage

The following processes help the individual stay consistent, build confidence, and respond to stress in healthier ways:

1. **Counterconditioning**

   Goal: Replace harmful stress responses (e.g., emotional eating, isolating, overworking) with healthier alternatives.

   - Practice mindfulness, deep breathing, or journaling instead of numbing or avoiding.
   - Use exercise or art as outlets for emotional stress.

2. **Stimulus control**

   Goal: Reduce or remove triggers that contribute to chronic stress.

   - Turn off phone notifications during downtime.
   - Create a calming bedtime routine to improve sleep.
   - Limit time with toxic relationships or stressful environments when possible.

3. **Helping relationships**

   Goal: Build a network of support and accountability.

   - Stay connected to a therapist, coach, or support group.
   - Check in regularly with a trusted friend or family member.
   - Ask for help when overwhelmed rather than going it alone.

4. **Reinforcement management**

   Goal: Use rewards to reinforce positive stress management behaviors.

- Treat yourself after a week of consistent meditation or movement.
- Celebrate non-scale victories, such as better sleep or fewer headaches.

5. **Self-liberation (ongoing commitment)**

   Goal: Strengthen the belief that stress can be managed and the person is in control.

   - Use affirmations or mantras such as "I am allowed to rest" or "I can create peace in my day."
   - Reflect on how far they've come: *"Three months ago I was having panic attacks. Now I take 10 minutes each day just to breathe."*

6. **Self-reevaluation**

   Goal: Reinforce alignment between their stress management actions and the person they want to be.

   - "I feel more like myself when I take time to decompress."
   - "I'm a better parent/partner when I take care of my mental health."

D. Health Literacy and Actioners

When a person is in the action phase of change, health literacy plays a critical role in their decision-making, which influences their ability to carry out and sustain their behavior change effectively. In the action phase, the person is *already doing the work*—now they need **clear, accurate, and actionable information** to do it **effectively and safely**. Without adequate health literacy, they may struggle to follow through on their plan correctly, make informed decisions, adjust when things don't go as expected and prevent relapse. Following are some important considerations related to health literacy for individuals in the action stage who may require additional attention and training:

Understanding how-to information: Comprehending instructions (e.g., medication use, exercise routines, meal plans) and reading labels, menus, prescriptions, or health monitoring tools (e.g., glucometers or fitness trackers) may require additional teaching/training.

Evaluating resources: Identifying reliable information (e.g., differentiating evidence-based guidance from myths or trends) is critical. This will facilitate making informed choices among treatment options, tools, or support groups.

Navigating the health system: Scheduling and attending appointments may require additional assistance.Communicating effectively with HCPs (e.g., asking questions, sharing concerns, reporting symptoms) may also be a skill that needs to be practiced and encouraged.

Making informed adjustments: Knowing how and when to modify behaviors based on results (e.g., changing diet if cholesterol remains high) and recognizing when professional guidance is needed may be a challenge.

Using digital tools: Accessing health portals, telehealth, or mobile apps may not be easy. Taking the time to ensure that reading and interpreting health data such as step counts, blood pressure logs, or calorie intake is understood may be required.

HCPs and educators can focus on the following when considering health literacy needs in the action phase:

- Use plain language and visual aids.
- Break information into small, actionable steps.
- Offer teach-back methods (e.g., "Can you tell me how you'll use this at home?").
- Provide multilingual or culturally relevant resources when needed.
- Encourage questions and help build confidence in decision-making.

Summary

In summary, this phase is where the hard work of sustaining new behaviors begins. Supporting a patient in the action phase of behavior change involves actively reinforcing their efforts, offering tools and strategies to facilitate the change, and creating an environment where they feel supported in maintaining those changes. People in the action phase need continued support to help them move toward maintenance, where the behavior change becomes a stable part of their routine. Recognize their commitment and acknowledge and reinforce their effort and progress, regardless of how small. Provide practical and step-by-step guidance with a focus on clear and actionable instructions. Avoid overwhelming them with too much information at once.

Support skill-building by teaching coping strategies, problem-solving, and behavior-specific skills (e.g., meal planning, stress management). This will help them prepare for real-life challenges and triggers. Encourage self-monitoring and SMART goal setting. In the action phase, it's essential to set goals that are manageable and that the patient feels confident they can achieve. There are thousands of apps available online, many of which are free. These will help in tracking their behavior, help with understanding the why, and increase their self-efficacy (which is paramount for sustained behavior change). Additionally, fostering a supportive environment is significant in this stage. Online or in-person support networks (e.g., family, friends, community), coaching, or other supportive services will help maintain the change and deal with relapse.

People with higher health literacy can better understand treatment options, resources, and consequences of different actions. They're more likely to evaluate the credibility of sources. They're better equipped to find and use services (e.g., hotlines, clinics, support groups). Health-literate individuals can ask better questions during appointments and clearly express concerns or needs. They're also more comfortable discussing sensitive topics such as trauma, depression, or medication. With good health literacy, people can anticipate setbacks and plan solutions, increasing their chances of sticking with the change.

Setbacks can occur, but resilience helps people stay on track. Discuss signs of slipping and how to take corrective action early. Normalize the struggle and frame it as part of the process. Remind patients to be kind to themselves if they don't always meet their goals. Avoid punishment or guilt-based tactics. Don't forget to celebrate success. Recognize and reinforce even small wins to build confidence and maintain momentum. These critical questions are designed to help the patient reflect on their current progress, identify challenges, and strengthen their commitment to lasting behavior change. They also help HCPs assess self-efficacy, adjust plans, and reinforce motivation for long-term success. By asking these questions regularly, HCPs can offer continuous support and facilitate the transition to the maintenance stage and sustaining changes long-term.

Critical Thinking Questions When Working With Someone in the Action Phase

Progress and commitment: These questions help assess the patient's emotional response to their behavior change, provide an opportunity to validate their efforts, and may offer an opportunity to discuss strategies for boosting confidence.

- *How are you feeling about the changes you've made so far? What positive changes have you noticed since you started working on this goal? How confident are you in your ability to keep up with this change?*

Challenges and obstacles: Identifying obstacles allows for problem-solving and helps address barriers to success.

- *What challenges have you encountered while trying to make these changes? Is there anything that is making it hard to stick to your new routine? How do you cope with situations that make it hard for you to stay on track?*

Support system: These help identify external sources of support that are playing a role in the patient's success and determine whether additional resources or connections are needed.

- *Who or what has helped you stay motivated during this process? Do you feel like you have enough support from others in this process?*

Reflection and motivation: These questions help the patient reflect on their intrinsic motivation and the deeper reasons behind their efforts. They also may encourage the patient to think about the potential consequences of not maintaining the change, which can reinforce their commitment to the new behavior.

- *Why is this change important to you? What motivates you to keep going, especially when things get difficult? What would happen if you stopped working toward this goal?*

Goal-setting and adjustments: These questions help the patient set new goals and keep them focused on forward progress.

- *What's your next goal or milestone in this process? Is there anything you would like to adjust in your current plan to make it easier or more effective?*

Self-monitoring and accountability: These encourage the patient to engage in self-monitoring, which helps them stay accountable and recognize their progress. These questions help the patient prepare for potential setbacks and encourage them to develop strategies to overcome them.

- *How do you track your progress? What is your plan if you encounter setbacks or challenges?*

Maintaining behavior change: These questions prompt the patient to think about sustainability and how they can maintain the behavior changes over time.

- *How do you plan to keep these changes going long-term? What are some of the things that help you stay motivated in the long run?*

Assessing external influences: This question helps identify external influences, such as work stress, family commitments, or environmental factors, that may affect the patient's ability to stay on track.

- *Are there any external factors that are making it easier or harder for you to maintain these changes?*

Reflecting on self-efficacy and confidence: These questions help the patient reflect on their strengths and reinforce their self-efficacy and autonomy in their behavior change journey.

- *What part of this process makes you feel most confident in your ability to succeed? Do you feel you are in control of your behavior change? Why or why not?*

Future outlook: This question encourages the patient to envision a future in which the change is permanent, helping solidify the behavior as part of their routine.

- *How do you see yourself maintaining this change in the future?*

Chapter 6

Maintenance

In this chapter, we will review which types of characteristics you might see in a patient who is trying to maintain the changes they have made. We will review the kinds of comments you might hear and how you might consider responding. Upon completion of this chapter, you should be able to identify when a patient is in the maintenance stage and the health education that would best match their needs.

Objectives

1. List key characteristics of someone in the maintenance stage.
2. Explain the appropriate health education for this stage.
3. Understand the relevance of health literacy.

Key Terms

- **Relapse prevention**
- **Ongoing motivation**
- **Lifestyle integration**

Scenario Description

John is a 58-year-old man who was diagnosed with hypertension three years ago. After being prescribed medication for his high blood pressure, he initially struggled with remembering to take his medications consistently and understanding the importance of long-term adherence.

However, after several doctor visits and education about the risks of uncontrolled hypertension (e.g., heart disease and stroke), John began to make a commitment to his health. For the past six months, he has been consistently taking his prescribed medication and making efforts to maintain his overall health. He has successfully integrated medication adherence into his daily routine and adopted other lifestyle changes, such as diet modification and regular physical activity.

Health status: Obese, with a body mass index of 40. Has sedentary job but walks daily.

A. Overview: Maintenance

Characteristics of the Stage

The maintenance phase in the transtheoretical model (TTM) is when an individual has successfully sustained behavior change for an extended period (usually six months or longer) and is working to maintain that change over the long term. The new behavior is part of their routine and has become more automatic or habitual. The focus shifts from making the change to keeping it going and preventing relapse. Although relapse can still occur, individuals in the maintenance phase have developed strategies to minimize the risk of returning to old habits. They are aware of potential triggers or situations in which they may be at risk of relapse and have coping strategies in place. Regular monitoring and assessment continue to ensure that progress is maintained.

Following are key characteristics of the maintenance stage:

- **Increased confidence and self-efficacy:** The person has greater self-efficacy (belief in their ability to sustain the behavior) and confidence in their ability to continue managing their condition. They feel empowered by their success and are motivated to continue their new behaviors.
- **Long-term focus:** The focus shifts from short-term goals to long-term health maintenance. The individual begins to recognize that

sustaining behavior change is a lifelong commitment and may take proactive measures to prevent setbacks.

- **Relapse prevention:** Situations or triggers that may lead to relapse are identified and understood (e.g., stress, busy schedules, changes in lifestyle), and there is a plan in place to work through the obstacles.

Healthcare providers (HCPs) and educators play a key role in helping patients sustain their behavior changes and avoid relapse. Reinforce the positive behavior by celebrating individual achievements and progress, recognizing that they have made a sustained effort. Commend the individual for their consistent adherence to medication, lifestyle changes, and/or self-management. Teach about the importance of continuing their behavior changes long-term, even when they feel well. It is important to emphasize that chronic conditions require ongoing management, as some might feel once goals are met or chronic conditions are controlled, they can stop some of the changes that have been made. Regularly update patients on the latest research, treatment guidelines, and strategies for maintaining their health.

Patient Conversations: Things You Might Hear the Patient Say

HCP: Good to see you, John. I reviewed your blood pressure logs—your readings have been stable for several months now. That's excellent progress [*praise*].

Patient in maintenance: Thanks! I've been keeping up with the walking every morning and sticking to the low-sodium diet. I also haven't missed a dose of my medication in over six months.

HCP: That's fantastic. It sounds like these habits are really becoming part of your daily life [*positive affirmation*].

Patient in maintenance: Yeah, it's just part of the routine now. I feel a lot better overall, too—more energy, sleeping better.

HCP: That's great to hear. This is exactly what we hope for in the maintenance phase—you're managing your health consistently. Have you run into any challenges keeping up with your routine [*exploring triggers/relapse prevention*]?

Patient in maintenance: Not really. I did have one weekend where I ate out more than usual, and my blood pressure was a bit higher, but I got right back on track the next week.

In this example, John has been able to maintain sustained changed for a significant period of time. The provider has acknowledged his success, praised his adherence to his medication regime, and helped him understand how this has improved his health outcomes. Although there was a slip-up that John acknowledged, the provider should not berate or provide negative reinforcement but instead praise him for getting back on track.

B. Health Education for Maintenance

In the maintenance stage of change, health education should focus on long-term success, relapse prevention, and continued growth. The person has already adopted healthy behaviors, so the goal now is to reinforce, support, and deepen those habits.Following are some key elements of health education that may be beneficial for people in this stage as well as examples of what the HCP or educator might say as a continuation of the patient-provider example that was reviewed earlier.

Reinforce positive behavior: Celebrate the patient's achievements and progress, recognizing that they've made a sustained effort. Positive reinforcement encourages continued commitment.

> *"Your blood pressure has remained stable for the past six months, and your commitment to your medication regimen is really paying off. Great job!"*

Educate regarding relapse prevention: Teach how to recognize the early warning signs of backsliding and facilitate the development of a personal relapse prevention plan. Emphasize that lapses are normal and manageable—not failure.

> *"It is great that you we aware of what you did that affected your blood pressure. No one is perfect, and you did the right thing by getting back on track the following week."*

> *"Even though you're feeling better, it's important to continue taking your medication to prevent future complications, like stroke or heart disease. Let's talk about those signs/ symptoms."*

<u>Develop coping strategies for stress or triggers:</u> Collaborate with patients to develop strategies for coping with potential setbacks. Encourage them to seek support when needed and remind them that lapses are normal but don't signal failure. Teach how to manage new or unexpected stressors without reverting to old behaviors.

> *"Sometimes meal prepping can help with ensuring we stick to our food goals. What other strategies are you using to track your food intake?"*

> *"Have you considered joining a support group for people managing hypertension? It could be helpful to connect with others who are going through the same experience."*

<u>Help sustain motivation:</u> Provide education on setting new, meaningful goals (e.g., increasing intensity of exercise, improving diet variety). Encourage journaling or self-reflection to track personal growth.

> *"Would you be interested in setting any new goals? Maybe incorporating some strength training or cutting back on caffeine?"*

"You've done an excellent job with medication adherence and healthy eating. Now, let's set a goal for increasing your daily physical activity to help keep your blood pressure within the ideal range."

Plan for the future: Teach how to adjust habits with life transitions (e.g., aging, job changes, travel). Prepare them for maintaining health during holidays, stress, or disruptions.

"You have done a great job maintaining these changes. I know you have some travel planned in the upcoming months. How are you going to ensure that you stick to your routine while you are away?"

"In the past, your job has gotten stressful during the holidays. Have you thought about ways to try to decrease that stress so that your blood pressure is not affected?"

During this phase, ensuring that individuals feel confident in their self-monitoring skills (e.g., blood pressure, weight, glucose) and understand how to adjust behaviors based on changes or new data is important. Keep them informed of new guidelines, treatments, or tools that support their health condition, understanding that some may need help with evaluating health information critically (health literacy reinforcement). Encourage lifestyle expansion by promoting cross-over behaviors (e.g., someone who started walking might now try yoga or strength training). This is the perfect time to introduce healthy changes in other areas, such as sleep hygiene or alcohol use.

Encourage individuals to maintain or build social support, such as family members, friends, or support groups. Social support can provide motivation and accountability. Suggest community programs, support groups, or online resources that provide ongoing education and motivation. They may be ready to advocate for health in community settings as well, which can then support others in their health journeys.

Reinforce communication skills with HCPs (e.g., asking questions, reporting changes).

Even in the maintenance phase, HCPs should monitor for any emerging complications or changes in the patient's condition. Therefore, the importance of regular follow-up visits should be stressed to track progress, provide reinforcement, and adjust treatment plans if necessary. Consistent visits can also help people to reflect on why they made the change in the first place and align their current behaviors with their personal values and life goals. Understand that this phase can still come with challenges, such as emotional ups and downs. Acknowledge those feelings without judgment and offer emotional support. If the person experiences emotional or mental health challenges related to their condition (e.g., anxiety about health), provide or refer for appropriate mental health support.

C. Key Processes of Change for the Maintenance Stage

The following processes help the individual reinforce healthy routines, adapt over time, and manage setbacks effectively:

1. **Self-reevaluation (ongoing identity shift)**

   Goal: Reinforce how their behavior reflects the person they want to be, such as in the following ways:

   - Saying, "I'm someone who takes care of my heart health"
   - Journaling or reflecting on how their lifestyle aligns with long-term values such as being active for their children or aging well

2. **Counterconditioning (habit strengthening)**

   Goal: Continue using healthy alternatives instead of old behaviors, such as the following:

- Choosing walking or yoga instead of watching television to unwind
- Preparing low-sodium meals rather than eating takeout
- Practicing deep breathing when feeling stressed instead of emotional eating

3. **Stimulus control**

   Goal: Maintain an environment that supports blood pressure control, such as in the following ways:

   - Keeping medication in a visible spot as a reminder
   - Meal prepping to avoid unhealthy food choices during the week
   - Scheduling blood pressure checks or check-ins as part of a routine

4. **Reinforcement management**

   Goal: Use positive reinforcement to maintain motivation, such as in the following ways:

   - Celebrating consistent blood pressure readings with nonfood rewards (e.g., getting a massage, a new book, a new pair of sneakers)
   - Setting new health-related goals (e.g., improving fitness level or sleep hygiene)

5. **Helping relationships**

   Goal: Sustain supportive connections that encourage a healthy lifestyle, such as in the following ways:

   - Continuing to engage with a provider, support group, or health coach
   - Encouraging family members to join in on healthy activities such as cooking or walking together

6. **Consciousness raising**

   Goal: Stay informed and aware of health updates and risks, such as in the following ways:

   - Learning about new hypertension guidelines or monitoring technologies
   - Understanding the impact of aging, stress, or other conditions on blood pressure

D. Health Literacy and Maintenance

When someone is in the maintenance phase, health literacy becomes a key tool for sustaining positive behavior and preventing relapse. At this point, they've already made a health-related change—now they're trying to stick with it. Health literacy in this stage is about empowering people to maintain, adapt, and grow their health behaviors through ongoing understanding, self-management, and informed decision-making. The following demonstrate how health literacy matters in that process:

Understanding long-term health needs: Health-literate individuals are better able to comprehend chronic or ongoing care—whether that's trauma recovery, mental health support, or stress management. They know why continued action is necessary, even when the problem seems to have passed.

Interpreting setbacks: A person with good health literacy can recognize that a slip (e.g., reconnecting with a toxic person, skipping a therapy session) doesn't mean total failure. They can analyze what happened, identify triggers, and adjust their approach.

Staying informed and adaptive: Health literacy helps people keep up with new information, resources, or strategies. They can critically evaluate what's useful and adapt their routines if needed—such as by switching providers, using new apps, or seeking alternative therapies.

Communicating ongoing needs: They're more likely to speak up when something isn't working or when they need support. That includes following up with health professionals, asking questions, and knowing how to navigate systems effectively (e.g., legal, medical, social services).

Building confidence and independence: Health literacy promotes self-efficacy—the belief that they can maintain change. It empowers people to own their journey, problem-solve, and continue making informed choices.

Summary

In summary, when someone is in the maintenance phase of behavior change, they've already made a health-related change and are working to sustain it long-term. At this stage, health education should focus on reinforcement, relapse prevention, and long-term self-management. Relapse prevention education should include teaching warning signs of setbacks and providing tools for coping with triggers, emotional stress, or social pressure. Encourage building a safety net of support groups and community connections.

Empowering the individual includes building communication skills, conflict resolution, stress management and mindfulness practices. Promotion of healthy routines (e.g., nutrition, exercise, and sleep) as part **lifestyle integration** in also a critical part of this phase. Tone matters, too: In the maintenance phase, education should feel encouraging, collaborative, and strength-based—less about risk and more about empowerment and sustainability. Normalize the ups and downs of healing and wellness. Continue to reinforce that needing help again is not failure—it's part of growth.

The maintenance phase is about keeping the momentum going—celebrating success, providing continuous education, and ensuring that the individual feels supported and motivated to sustain healthy behaviors for the long term. The critical thinking questions in the following section can help assess progress, encourage reflection, and reinforce commitment to sustained behavior change. By asking these critical questions, HCPs and educators can help individuals in this phase feel supported, confident, and equipped to continue their behavior changes long-term. These critical questions not only reinforce the person's progress but also provide **ongoing motivation** and solutions for potential challenges.

Critical Thinking Questions When Working With Someone in the Maintenance Phase

Reflecting on progress: This helps the individual reflect on the long-term benefits of the change, boosts confidence, and reinforces tangible benefits of their efforts.

- *What are you most proud of regarding the changes you've made? What impact have these changes had on your daily life or overall well-being? How have you felt since making these changes?*

Identifying challenges and barriers: This encourages the individual to reflect on how they've managed potential relapses and boosts their sense of resilience and control. Understanding stressors or triggers can help anticipate challenges and develop strategies to deal with them effectively.

- *Are there any situations that are making it harder to stick to your new routine? How have you handled any setbacks or temptations to return to old habits?*

Reinforcing motivation and self-efficacy: Understanding intrinsic motivations can help reinforce the long-term commitment to the new behavior and align it with personal values. It will also reinforce the person's sense of purpose and the value of maintaining their change over time.

- *What motivates you to continue maintaining this change? What keeps you focused on your goals despite life's challenges?*

Tracking and monitoring progress: Encouraging ongoing self-monitoring reinforces accountability and allows for early detection of any issues.

- *How do you continue to track your progress, and what tools do you use to stay on track? Do you feel like you're making steady progress, or is there anything you'd like to adjust?*

Long-term sustainability and lifestyle integration: These encourage the person to think about how the behavior has become part of their identity and daily life, making it easier to continue without effort. Identifying difficulties in daily routines can help make adjustments to improve long-term adherence.

- *How can you integrate these changes into your lifestyle so that they become a permanent part of your routine? Are there any habits or routines that are still difficult to maintain, and how can we work to make them easier?*

Preparing for setbacks and relapse prevention: This helps the person anticipate potential triggers and plan for setbacks, making it easier to stay on track. Encourages resilience by helping the individual prepare mentally and emotionally for challenges.

- *What could cause you to fall back into old habits, and how can we plan to avoid or handle these situations? If you did experience a setback, how would you handle it, and what steps would you take to get back on track? Do you have any strategies in place to deal with stress or changes in your routine that could affect your progress?*

Looking ahead and anticipating future goals: This encourages long-term vision and motivates continued progress, helping the individual see their behavior changes as part of a lifelong commitment to health. It also helps the person focus on further growth and sets the stage for new goals, preventing complacency.

- *How do you see yourself in the next six months to a year regarding your health and well-being? What other health or lifestyle goals would you like to work on now that you've successfully maintained this change?*

Conclusion

Health education is the foundation of behavior change. Without understanding *what* to change, *why* it matters, and *how* to do it, people are far less likely to act—or sustain it over time. Most preventable illnesses—such as heart disease, diabetes, and hypertension—are closely linked to behaviors such as poor diet, physical inactivity, smoking, and medication nonadherence. Helping individuals with behavior change is essential to improving health outcomes and reducing the burden of chronic disease and should be considered a primary role of all healthcare professionals.

Health education drives behavior change by helping individuals recognize the link between their behavior and health outcomes. If done properly, health education turns vague advice, such as "Eat healthier," into specific, actionable knowledge (e.g., "Reducing the amount of salt in your meals will decrease blood pressure"). People need guidance on how to make a change, not just on why it's important. Health education provides a clear roadmap and gives tools, skills, and step-by-step strategies to take meaningful action.

Why Does Proper Health Education Drive Behavior Change?

1. **Builds confidence (self-efficacy):** When people understand what they're doing and why, they feel more capable of making and maintaining the change. Proper education reduces fear, confusion, and helplessness.
2. **Supports long-term maintenance:** Health education should not be a one-time event. It equips people with skills for lifelong self-

management and helps individuals adapt to new challenges and prevent relapse.

3. **Addresses misconceptions and misinformation:** It contests myths, stigma, and/or culturally held beliefs that may block change. Accurate health education helps people make informed, empowered decisions.
4. **Improves communication and engagement:** When people are well informed, they can actively participate in care decisions and discussions with providers. This enhances shared decision-making and trust in health care.

Remember, health literacy is the base of effective health education and successful chronic disease management. It determines whether people can truly understand, process, and act on the information they're given about their health.

Health Education Works Only if It's Understood

Even the best health education won't lead to change if it's too complex, full of jargon, or not culturally relevant. People with limited health literacy may:

- Misinterpret instructions
- Struggle with medication adherence
- Avoid follow-ups or screenings
- Be confused about symptoms or diagnoses

Chronic Diseases Require Active Self-Management

Conditions such as diabetes, hypertension, asthma, and heart disease require daily decisions and long-term behaviors, such as taking medications correctly; monitoring blood sugar or blood pressure; managing diet, activity, and symptoms; and knowing when to seek medical help. Without strong health literacy, patients can't manage these tasks reliably or safely.

Supports Better Communication and Shared Decision-Making

People with strong health literacy are more likely to ask questions, understand treatment options, express concerns clearly, and engage in shared decision-making. This leads to better adherence, higher satisfaction, and more personalized care.

Reduces Health Disparities

Populations with lower health literacy often face worse chronic disease outcomes and higher hospitalization rates. Improving health literacy is a health equity strategy—it helps close the gap for vulnerable and underserved groups.

Improves Outcomes and Lowers Costs

Better health literacy leads to fewer emergency department visits, lower hospitalization rates, better disease control, and fewer complications (Cho et al., 2008; Shahid et al., 2022). Educated, health-literate patients are more empowered to make cost-effective, prevention-focused decisions.

Health literacy is the key that unlocks the power of health education, especially in chronic disease management. Without it, patients are left confused and overwhelmed. With it, they become informed partners in their care, capable of making meaningful changes that improve their health and quality of life. Health literacy and health equity are deeply connected—both are essential to ensuring that every individual has a fair opportunity to achieve their best possible health. When people understand health information, they are more likely to access care, follow treatment plans, and make informed decisions. Without adequate health literacy, individuals may be left behind, especially those from underserved or marginalized communities.

Low health literacy is often a symptom of inequity. People with lower health literacy often face systemic barriers, including limited education, language differences, racism and discrimination, poverty, and lack of access to digital tools or quality care. These factors overlap with the social determinants of health, making low health literacy both a consequence and driver of health disparities (National Academies of Sciences, Engineering, and Medicine, 2017). Improving health literacy is a strategy for equity. As healthcare professionals we can improve health literacy by the following:

- Use plain language in materials and conversations.
- Provide interpreters and translated resources.
- Design and deliver culturally relevant and patient-centered health education.
- Teach individuals how to navigate the healthcare system and advocate for themselves.

When healthcare systems adapt to the needs of those with lower health literacy, everyone benefits—especially those at risk of being marginalized. Health literacy is not just an individual skill; it's also a system responsibility. Equitable systems are those that communicate clearly, reduce complexity, include diverse voices in care design, and proactively close gaps in access and understanding. **Health equity can't be achieved without addressing health literacy.** Ensuring that all people can understand, access, and use health information is key to removing barriers, reducing disparities, and creating a more just and inclusive healthcare system.

Key Reasons Behavior Change Support Matters

1. **Improves health outcomes**
    - Supporting lasting behavior change can lead to better disease control, fewer complications, and longer life.

2. **Empowers patients**
   - It builds patient confidence, self-management skills, and health literacy—so that patients can take control of their health.
3. **Reduces healthcare costs**
   - Preventing hospitalizations and emergency care through healthier behaviors reduces systemwide costs.
4. **Strengthens provider-patient relationships**
   - Helping with behavior change requires trust, communication, and shared decision-making—all of which improve care quality.
5. **Addresses root causes**
   - Treating symptoms alone isn't enough; lasting wellness requires addressing the underlying behaviors and lifestyle factors.
6. **Promotes long-term wellness**
   - Behavior change leads to healthier habits that benefit patients across their lifespan—not just in the short term.

Behavior change is the foundation of prevention, chronic disease management, and overall health. As a healthcare professional, guiding individuals through that change is one of the most impactful things you can do. ***Proper health education is not just about giving information—it's about empowering transformation.*** It's how people learn to take charge of their health, overcome barriers, and build habits that last.

References

Barnhart, C. (2020, June 19). *5 principles to motivational interviewing.* EMS1. https://www.ems1.com/ems-products/mobile-computers/articles/5-principles-to-motivational-interviewing-C6NBkSFwDPSLcI5L/

Brenan, M. & Jones, J. (2024, January 22) *Ethics ratings of nearly all professions down in U.S.* https://news.gallup.com/poll/608903/ethics-ratings-nearly-professions-down.aspx

Centers for Disease Control and Prevention. (2024a, October 4). *About chronic diseases.* https://www.cdc.gov/chronicdisease/index.htm

Centers for Disease Control and Prevention. (2024b, July 12). *Fast facts: Health and economic costs of chronic diseases.* https://www.cdc.gov/cbhronic-disease/data-research/facts-stats/?CDC_AAref_Val=https://www.cdc.gov/chronicdisease/about/costs/index.htm

Centers for Disease Control and Prevention. (2024c, May 15). *National diabetes statistics report.* https://www.cdc.gov/diabetes/php/data-research/index.html

Centers for Disease Control and Prevention. (2024d, May 14). *Adult obesity facts.* https://www.cdc.gov/obesity/adult-obesity-facts/index.html

Cho, Y., Lee, S. D., Arozullah, A. M., & Crittenden, K. S. (2008). Effects of health literacy on health status and health service utilization amongst the elderly. *Social Science & Medicine, 66*(8), 1809–1816.

Coughlin, S. S., Vernon, M., Hatzigeorgiou, C., & George, V. (2021). Health literacy, social determinants of health, and disease prevention and control. *Journal of Environmental Health Sciences, 6*(1), 3061–3065.

Division for Heart Disease and Stroke Prevention. (2023, May 12).*Estimated hypertension prevalence, treatment and control among U.S. adults.* https://millionhearts.hhs.gov/data-reports/hypertension-prevalence.html

Fixsen, D. L., Naoom, S. F., Blase, K. A., Friedman, R. M. & Wallace, F. (2005). *Implementation research: A synthesis of the literature.* University of South Florida, Louis de la Parte Florida Mental Health Institute, the National Implementation Research Network (FMHI Publication 231).

Miller, W. R., & Rollnick, S. (2013). *Motivational interviewing: Helping people change* (3rd ed.). Guilford Press.

Multiple Chronic Conditions Resource Center. (2025). *Multiple chronic conditions.* https://multiplechronicconditions.org/

National Academies of Sciences, Engineering, and Medicine. (2017). *Communities in action: Pathways to health equity.* National Academies Press. https://doi.org/10.17226/24624

National Cancer Institute. (2025). *Cancer stat facts: Common cancer sites.*https://seer.cancer.gov/statfacts/html/common.html

National Center for Health Statistics. (2025, December 30). *All ages deaths by multiple cause of death (2018–2023).* Mortality Data on CDC WONDER. https://wonder.cdc.gov/mcd.html

National Institutes of Health. (2025, February 21). *Plain language at NIH.* https://www.nih.gov/institutes-nih/nih-office-director/office-communications-public-liaison/clear-communication/plain-language-nih

NCD Alliance. (n.d.). *Chronic respiratory diseases.* https://ncdalliance.org/why-ncds/ncds/chronic-respiratory-diseases-0

Prochaska, J. O., & Velicer, W. F. (1997). The transtheoretical model of health behavior change. *American Journal of Health Promotion, 12*(1), 38–48. https://doi.org/10.4278/0890-1171-12.1.38

Shahid, R., Shoker, M., Chu, L. M., Frehlick, R., Ward, H., & Pahwa, P. (2022). Impact of low health literacy on patients' health outcomes: A multicenter cohort study. *BMC Health Services Research, 22*, 1148. https://doi.org/10.1186/s12913-022-08527-9

Index